The BMA Family Doctor Gu

**Arthritis**

CW00419215

*Titles in the series:*

*Confusion in Old Age*
*Gallstones and Liver Problems*
*Arthritis*
*Asthma*
*Children's Health 1–5*
*Strokes and their Prevention*

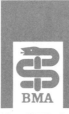

# FAMILY DOCTOR GUIDES

# Arthritis

## Prof. Paul Dieppe

Series editor: Dr Tony Smith

*Professor Dieppe is ARC Professor of Rheumatology at the Bristol Royal Infirmary.*

*Published by Equation in association with the British Medical Association*

First published 1988

Dieppe, P.A. (Paul Adrian)
    Arthritis.
    1. Man. Joints. Arthritis
    I. Title  II. Series
    616.7'22

    ISBN 1–85330–050–3

**Picture acknowledgements**

Arthritis Care: p. 47, 49, 113; Wellcome Institute Library, London:
p. 65; General Council & Register of Osteopaths: p.100; Disabled
Living Foundation: p.101; David Woodroffe: diagrams; Derek
Marriott: cartoons.

Equation, Wellingborough, Northamptonshire NN8 2RQ, England.

Typeset by Columns of Reading
Printed in Great Britain by The Bath Press, Avon

10  9  8  7  6  5  4  3  2  1

# Contents

1 ARTHRITIS AND RHEUMATISM    7
Understanding helps; Movement and the
'musculoskeletal system'; The structure and function
of joints; Fibrous joints; What are arthritis and
rheumatism?; Periarticular disorders; Articular
disorders; No need for gloom

2 WHO GETS ARTHRITIS?    14
How common is rheumatism?; How common is
arthritis?; Which types are most common?;
So who gets arthritis?

3 WHAT CAUSES ARTHRITIS?    19
What causes diseases in general?; Some factors in
arthritis; Susceptibility, triggers and progression

4 EFFECTS OF ARTHRITIS    25
Factors that determine effects of arthritis; The main
effects of arthritis

5 OSTEOARTHRITIS    31
Who gets osteoarthritis?; What causes osteoarthritis?;
How does it effect the joints?; Which joints are
affected?; Symptoms and signs; Complications;
What tests are helpful?; How is osteoarthritis treated?;
What can you expect?

6 RHEUMATOID ARTHRITIS    40
Who gets rheumatoid arthritis?; What causes
rheumatoid arthritis?; What happens in the joints?;
Symptoms and signs; Complications; What tests are
helpful?; How is rheumatoid arthritis treated?;
Outcome; Conclusion

7 ANKYLOSING SPONDYLITIS AND RELATED DISORDERS    53
Some explanation; Ankylosing spondylitis;
Reactive arthritis and Reiter's syndrome;
Psoriasis and arthritis; Colitis and arthritis

8  GOUT, PSEUDOGOUT AND JOINT CRYSTALS                    62
   Gout; Calcium crystals: pseudogout and related
   diseases

9  SOME UNCOMMON FORMS OF ARTHRITIS                       69
   Connective tissue diseases; Joint infections;
   Tumours (cancer) in joints; Bone and collagen
   diseases, and other miscellaneous causes of
   arthritis; So what?

10 PERIARTICULAR DISORDERS AND BACK PAIN                  75
   Periarticular disorders; Some periarticular disorders;
   Back pain; Painful but not life-threatening!

11 CHILDHOOD AND OLD AGE                                  83
   Arthritis in children; Arthritis in the elderly

12 CAN ARTHRITIS BE TREATED?                              86
   Remission; An age-old problem; Aims and objectives;
   Types of treatment available

13 DRUGS, INJECTIONS AND THERAPISTS                       91
   About drugs; Pain killers; Anti-inflammatory agents;
   Steroids; Disease-modifying agents; Problems and
   responsibility; Injections; The therapists

14 SURGERY                                               102
   Which diseases might need surgery?; What types
   of operation are there?; Which joints can be
   operated on?; When is surgery recommended?

15 ALTERNATIVE COMPLEMENTARY MEDICINE                    107
   Differences between traditional and alternative
   medicine; Special problems in arthritis; Alternative
   therapies related to conventional medicine;
   Treatments not used with conventional medicine;
   Conclusions

16 SELF-HELP AND LIVING WITH DISABILITY                  112
   Becoming an 'arthritic'; Relaxation; Joint protection;
   Rest and exercise; Your home, garden, work and
   sport; Common questions and problems

USEFUL ADDRESSES                                         123

INDEX                                                    125

# 1 Arthritis and rheumatism

Most of us take for granted our ability to move about as we like and without pain. But people with arthritis and rheumatism are not so lucky. Their disorders limit what they can do, and they may make everyday living a painful experience.

## Understanding helps

One of the best ways of coping with any disorder is to understand it better. Some knowledge of what is going on and why often makes it obvious how to improve the situation. Knowing what could or won't happen makes it easier to face the future. Arthritis may be rather unpredictable but we do know a good deal about it, including the fact that it often improves spontaneously. The aim of this book is to help sufferers understand more about arthritis, in the hope that this will make it easier for them, and their friends and relatives, to cope.

Before considering what goes wrong and how arthritis and rheumatism develop, it is useful to look at the normal functioning of the body structures that enable us to move around.

## Movement and the 'musculoskeletal system'

For normal movement we need bones, muscles and joints – the three main components of the *musculoskeletal system*. The bones are our body's scaffolding; they provide rigidity and form to our trunk and limbs. The muscles contract forcefully to produce movement. The joints are the hinges between our bones and their job is to allow us to move parts of our body smoothly and steadily – joints have to provide some stability as well as mobility.

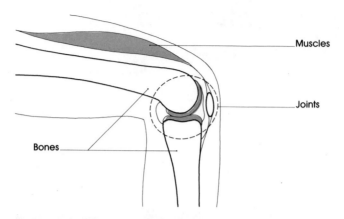

Muscles

Joints

Bones

**The three components of the muscoloskeletal system.**

## Well designed

The musculoskeletal system serves a mechanical function – it lets us move around. But, like any other complicated mechanical system, such as a car, efficient, trouble-free performance depends on good design, faultless components and careful use. A badly designed car or one containing faulty components will let you down however carefully you drive. Conversely, the best car in the world won't survive intact if you drive it into a brick wall. It's the same with bones, muscles and joints. Severe injury will break bones (fractures); tear muscles, ligaments and tendons (strains and sprains); and damage joints. A few of us develop diseases early in our lives that damage the system. Age may also take its toll, causing older people to slow up and get more than their fair share of pain. But the design and components of the musculoskeletal system are so good that most of us can continue to lead active, mobile lives for a good deal longer than the lifespan of several average cars.

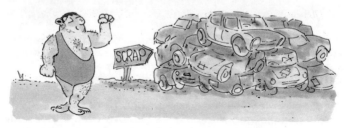

*Humans go on working longer than cars.*

## The structure and function of joints

Our joints are beautifully designed mechanical devices. The main components of the joints between limb bones (which are known as the synovial joints) include the shaped bone ends, a smooth covering of cartilage, and a thin surrounding membrane.

### Bone

The shape of the bone ensures that the two halves of the joint fit together and can move in some directions but not others. Some joints, such as the knee and elbow, are like hinges, allowing only one type of movement. Others, the shoulder and hip, for example, are designed like a ball and socket, providing a wide range of free movements. Bones are living tissues, strengthened by mineral, and they can change shape and form if they are under abnormal stress or damaged by diseases like arthritis.

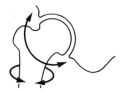

1. Ball and socket joints, like the hip, can move in many directions.

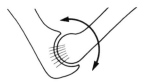

2. Hinge joints, like the elbow, only move in one direction. Ligaments as well as bone shape stops them from moving in other planes.

### Cartilage

Cartilage is a layer of glistening, tough 'gristle', attached to the bone end. It acts as a shock absorber but also allows smooth, gliding movement between the two bone ends. In fact there is less friction between the two cartilage surfaces in a joint than there is between a skate on ice. Some complex joints, like the knee, contain extra pads of cartilage. The proper name for these cartilages is the menisci and they are prone to injury, which is why so many sportsmen and women have problems with their knees. Unfortunately cartilage is not very good at repairing itself if it has been badly damaged.

## Membranes

The membrane surrounding a joint is known as the synovium. It produces a small amount of a sticky liquid, called synovial fluid, which helps lubricate the joint and also provides nutrition for the cartilage. The synovial membrane can easily become inflamed and may then produce extra fluid, of the wrong consistency.

## Capsule

The synovium is covered on the outside by a thicker membrane, the capsule, which surrounds ('encapsulates') the joint.

## Ligaments

In some joints the capsule is thickened and toughened by strong fibres which control the range of joint movement and help provide stability. These are the ligaments.

## Muscles, tendons and bursae

Outside the capsule of the joint are muscles, tendons, bursae and soft tissue. Muscles are attached to bones by tendons. The tendons usually run over the surface of a joint, and are attached close to its edge, so that maximum leverage can be

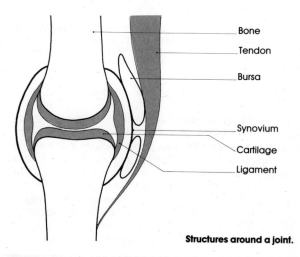

Bone

Tendon

Bursa

Synovium

Cartilage

Ligament

**Structures around a joint.**

applied. Bursae are small fluid-filled sacs that help reduce friction if the tendons and bones are rubbing over each other or when they are very close to the surface skin. Tendons and ligaments are easily injured and are often torn or damaged where they join a bone. A bursa, like the synovium, is prone to inflammation and can swell up with excess fluid.

## Fibrous joints

Some of the joints in the spine, skull and chest wall are not the same as the synovial joints so far described – they occur where much less movement is needed between the individual bones. These are the fibrous joints. They consist of a pad of cartilage between the bones and have no joint cavity. The cartilage pad has more give in it than the bone and allows a small amount of movement; it also acts as an effective shock absorber. The inter-vertebral joints in the spine are good examples of fibrous joints.

## What are arthritis and rheumatism?

The word arthritis literally means inflammation in a joint but it has come to be used for any type of joint disease. Rheumatism is an even less clearcut term, used to describe pain coming from the joints or the structures around them including muscles. Anything that damages the joints will also affect the nearby bone and muscles. Similarly, disorders affecting any of the structures near a joint can cause the same sort of problems as arthritis. So the terms 'arthritis' and 'rheumatism' cover quite a wide range of disorders. Furthermore, there are many different types of arthritis; almost as many as the number of different joints in the body – about 200 in both cases. Some are severe, many are mild. Some get worse, many get better.

> **When someone tells you they have arthritis, it could mean a lot of different things.**

### The different types of arthritis

Although some 200 different types of arthritis have been described, they can all be classified into a few different groups. The first division is between diseases of the joint itself (articular disorders) and those affecting mainly surrounding tissues such as tendons, ligaments or bursae (periarticular disorders).

## Periarticular disorders

Periarticular disorders are the most common. Many are caused by overuse or minor injury and most get better after a while. They include inflammation of bursae, such as 'housemaid's knee'; damage to the insertion of tendons into bone, as in 'tennis elbow'; and torn ligaments, for example a sprained ankle. Most of these conditions occur singly, causing pain in only one spot. It may be difficult, however, for the sufferer to be sure where the pain is coming from. The pain may spread all round the area, even if it originates from a small part. Many forms of low back pain are caused by damage to single periarticular areas in the spine, but the pain may spread widely, even going into the buttocks and legs.

### 'Fibrositis'

'Fibrositis' is another type of periarticular disorder. It is also known as muscular rheumatism, and is pain coming from one or more areas of muscle around the joints. Fibrositis is sometimes more widespread than other forms of periarticular rheumatism, and can affect several different parts of the body at the same time. None of these periarticular disorders is dangerous or causes permanent damage, and treatment is often simple and effective. They are discussed more fully on p. 75.

## Articular disorders

Articular disorders, arthritis, can also be subdivided into a few main categories. The main distinction is into:

- Diseases that cause inflammation affecting mainly the synovium;
- Osteoarthritis, which damages the surface cartilage and underlying bone.

There are many different types of inflammatory disease of joints, including those caused by infections, those triggered by crystals (such as gout), and distinctive generalised joint diseases such as rheumatoid arthritis and ankylosing spondylitis. The main categories will be described more in later chapters.

## No need for gloom

Some people with arthritic diseases become severely disabled by joint damage, but fortunately they are in the minority. Many get a lot of pain, at least for a few months or years, but even the worst forms of arthritis often improve with time, lessening the pain and stiffness and allowing the sufferer to adapt, adjust and improve the quality of life. The various treatments described later usually help relieve the symptoms and sometimes provide dramatic relief, and there are also many ways in which those who suffer from arthritis can help themselves. There is therefore no need for gloom, despondency or a negative attitude, even if you know you have a serious form of arthritis.

# 2 Who gets arthritis?

We all get aches and pains in our muscles and joints from time to time, perhaps after sitting or lying awkwardly or after uaccustomed exercise. These aches don't mean that there is anything wrong; they are caused by normal stresses and strains we put on our muscles and joints. They may be at their worst when we are tired, depressed, or have some other illness such as the 'flu. They can vary a lot in how painful they are and how much they affect us, but are usually no more than an occasional nuisance.

## How common is rheumatism?

As many as half of the population will suffer at some time from periarticular rheumatism in one form or another. These very common problems occur most often in young and middle-aged adults, and in those who put a lot of stress on their joints. Some people seem to be more prone than others, and may get several episodes of tennis elbow or shoulder pains. The pain is variable and generally felt in only one area. The effects depend on the site and on the person with the problem. A tennis elbow, for example will be much more worrying for the professional tennis player than for his footballing friend. These very common disorders don't normally cause any permanent pain, damage or disability. They are discussed more on p. 76.

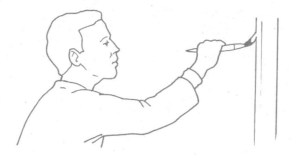

*An elbow disorder matters a lot to a painter.*

## How common is arthritis?

Arthritis affects something like one in every five or ten people. About 200 different types have been identified but most of them are rare; the few common forms are discussed in greater detail in other parts of this book.

Arthritis is no respecter of age, sex, race, colour or creed. It is found throughout the world, although the type, severity and consequences vary in different countries and cultures. As the population of the western world gets generally healthier and lives longer, arthritis becomes a more important cause of disability.

The effects of arthritis depend very much on the type of disease as well as the sufferer. Many forms are relatively mild, no more than a nuisance, but others can cause severe pain, deformity and disability.

---

**The total cost of arthritis to the community, as well as to the individual, is now enormous.**

---

### A burden on the community

Many people put up with pain and problems without complaining much or going to their doctor. Indeed many elderly people regard things like rheumatism as a part of being old! People are increasingly health conscious, however, and more of us are now looking for help and solutions to arthritis and rheumatism where previously we would have been prepared to 'grin and bear it'.

One way of getting an idea of the size of the problem is by checking on the reasons for people consulting their general practitioner.

---

**Surveys have shown that between one in five and one in ten of all visits to GPs are caused by arthritis and rheumatism.**

---

The commonest causes of visits to the GP are pain in the back or neck; periarticular rheumatism around the shoulders, elbows, knees and other joints; and osteoarthritis. Relatively few of those who go to their GP, however, are subsequently referred to a hospital specialist.

## A major health-care problem

The burden on society can be judged from the amount of lost working time or the number of disabled people requiring help. One recent survey showed that in Britain alone over 60 million lost working days each year are caused by arthritis, representing a cash value in excess of £1000 million. In addition, about one third of all severely disabled people have an arthritic cause of their incapacity.

The cash value of the disablement is hard to compute, but enormous. The burden of suffering for those with these diseases, as well as for those who care for them, is incalculable.

**Arthritis is rapidly becoming one of the major health-care problems of our time.**

## The effects of age and sex

The different forms of arthritis tend to occur most at certain times of life, and often have a predilection for either men or women. Gout, for example, is largely a disease of middle-aged men, whereas rheumatoid arthritis affects young or middle-aged women the most. The overall figure for the numbers of people with arthritis (that is, between one in five and one in ten) masks the fact that children get a few special types only, and that men tend to suffer from different forms of arthritis from women.

## Why these differences?

The reasons for these differences are complex and not fully understood. We do know, however, that the body's defence mechanisms change as we grow up and get older. We also know that the ageing process affects joints and how they adapt to injury. Finally, sex hormones also help control joint function and influence the type and severity of disease. Whatever the reasons, the common rheumatic diseases can be split up into groups according to the age group and sex they are most likely to affect, as shown in the table.

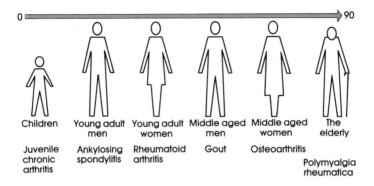

## Which types are most common?

Osteoarthritis is the most common form of arthritis. It affects women more than men, and generally occurs in the middle-aged and elderly. Rheumatoid arthritis also has a preference for women, but often starts in younger people whereas gout and ankylosing spondylitis are both more common in young men. There is one special form of arthritis, juvenile chronic arthritis, that occurs only in children. Other diseases of the musculoskeletal system, such as pseudogout and polymyalgia rheumatica, are largely confined to the elderly.

## So who gets arthritis?

These facts and figures still don't answer the question, who will get arthritis? Unfortunately, there is no way of telling who will and who won't suffer from it. Some forms run in families, but most don't. The causes, discussed in the next chapter, are not fully understood, so it is hard to pinpoint things that people do that will or won't lead to arthritis.

> **Normal, hard activity is not the cause of arthritis.**

On the positive side, however, we know that full active use of our bodies and their joints is good for our health. Furthermore, at least four out of every five of us, eating, drinking, sleeping and living our way through our varied lives, will never get any form of arthritis, however long we live.

# 3 What causes arthritis?

There is no single 'cause' of arthritis. Just as there are many different types of rheumatism and arthritis, there are also many different contributory factors.

## What causes diseases in general?

Diseases are either *congenital* or *acquired*. In other words, there are some diseases that people are born with and others that only develop during life. Most forms of arthritis come on during adult life and are therefore classified as acquired conditions.

Causes of disease

GENES                                    ENVIRONMENT

Variable body make-up          Injury, infection, etc.

DISEASE

An example: Fractures and bones

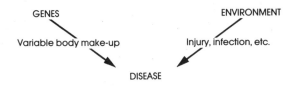

1. GENETIC  .

Born with thin bones

Multiple fractures without injury

2. ENVIRONMENTAL

Born with normal bones

Fracture after a motor-bike accident

3. MIXED

Born with a tendency to get thin bones in old age

Fracture after fall

## Genetic and environmental causes

Causes of disease can be divided into *genetic* and *environmental* factors. The genetic factors describe the influence of the genes in our body, which control our make-up.

Some people are born with a slight abnormality in one of their genes that can result in a deformity or other abnormality at birth (a congenital disease). But some inherited genetic defects matter only if the body is damaged in some other way. A crude example would be an inherited genetic tendency to grow small, thin bones. If this were severe, bones might break during normal usage, and the disease would be apparent at, or shortly after, birth. If the defect were milder, however, it might never matter and never be noticed. Alternatively, some bones might break more easily than normal so that a series of fractures in adult life would lead to the realisation that there was a genetic problem. There is such a disease, called 'osteogenesis imperfecta', and the exact gene change and consequent bone abnormality is well understood.

Of course, most fractures are caused by injury and have nothing to do with abnormal bones. They are examples of environmental disease. But in some types of fractures – the broken hips that occur so often and so easily in elderly people – a combination of several different factors is to blame. The genetic make-up of different people controls, to some extent, how they age and how much their bones get thinner in later life. Several other factors, including weight, diet and smoking, activity and exercise, all affect the ageing of bones. Then there is the fall or other incident that 'causes' the fracture. These broken bones are a good example of a problem whose 'cause' is a complex interaction of several different genetic and environmental factors.

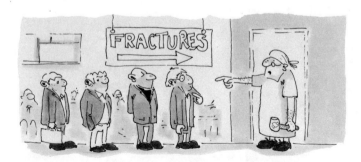

*Most fractures are caused by accidents.*

The reason for dwelling on the example of broken bones is twofold. First, most forms of arthritis are like the hip fractures of older people; they are caused by an interaction of many different factors rather than a single problem. Secondly, joints, like bones, are subject to injury and mechanical damage, which matters only if there is something else wrong with the system. Furthermore, bones and joints both grow, develop and age in a variable way, so that age and ageing have a great influence on the causes and type of disorder.

## Some factors in arthritis

Many different factors influence your chances of getting arthritis. In subsequent chapters the most important influences in each of the major diseases will be discussed, but this section provides a brief overview.

### Genetics and family susceptibility

Many forms of arthritis 'run in families', which means that relatives of sufferers may be more likely to get the disease than others. This is true of gout and ankylosing spondylitis, and, to a lesser extent, of rheumatoid and osteoarthritis. This tendency is

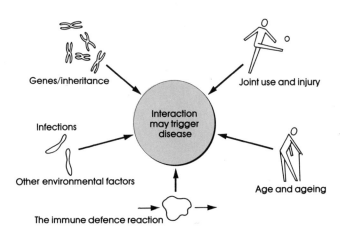

not, however, very strong. If the average chance of getting a particular type of arthritis (such as rheumatoid) were 1 in 100, it could double if there were a strong family history of the disease, but the chance then would still be only 2 in 100.

Researchers are now beginning to understand the genetic background to many of these diseases, explaining why they run in families. For example, the presence of a certain type of gene is known to increase the chance of getting ankylosing spondylitis about 100 fold. The challenge now is to understand how this operates. But however you look at it, genetics is not the whole story; it is a possible explanation for susceptibility, not the cause.

### Use and abuse of joints

Severe injuries to joints sometimes seem to lead to arthritis. This is less important than one might expect, although it is one of the factors in osteoarthritis particularly. In fact, normal use, including plenty of vigorous activity, seems to be good for joints.

Joint use and abuse will clearly affect the type and severity of disease in someone who has arthritis, but it is not very important as a cause.

### Obesity, diet and the weather

What we eat is often considered the root cause of all our ailments. In Britain we can also blame the weather. But arthritis occurs all over the world, in many different people, in many different climates, and irrespective of what people eat. Diet doesn't seem to have much to do with getting it. A few people with arthritis find that what they eat seems to alter the condition, but as with joint usage, this is more of an effect on the established disease than the cause. Similarly, being overweight puts stresses on joints, and will make it more difficult if you already have arthritis, but it probably won't have much effect on your chance of getting it. Damp weather may make damaged joints hurt more, but the weather doesn't cause the damage.

### Infection

Some forms of arthritis are clearly triggered off by an infection (see reactive arthritis, p. 58). This could be the case too in many other forms of the disease including ankylosing spondylitis and rheumatoid arthritis.

### Age and ageing

Different forms of arthritis occur in children, in young adults, and in the elderly. Growth, as well as ageing, affects the type of disease, as well as individual susceptibility to it. Growth and ageing are associated with subtle changes in the structure and function of joints, and they also affect the body's defence system.

### Immunology and the body's defences

Some types of arthritis are associated with abnormalities in the way in which the body defends itself against infection. This 'immunological system' involves a complex series of responses designed to protect the tissues from damage and disease. Occasionally, however, the system seems to attack the body instead of an invading organism – this is called 'autoimmunity'. In rheumatoid arthritis and many of the rarer forms of inflammatory joint diseases there is an element of autoimmunity, which may be very important in keeping these conditions going. It is unclear what leads to the autoimmunity in the first place, however, and how much of it is a result of these diseases rather than their cause.

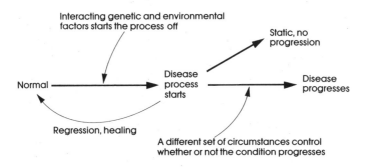

### Susceptibility, triggers and progression

The many different factors interact in the development of arthritic diseases. Some, like genetic make-up, affect susceptibility. Others, such as infections, may be trigger factors which start the diseases off.

> **Many quite different things can influence the way the disease develops and outcome of the arthritis once it has started.**

Most factors commonly blamed for 'causing' arthritis, including the weather, diet, stress, exercise, hormones and such like, have more to do with the pain and other effects of arthritis than they do with the fundamental causes. But current research on genetics, infective triggers, autoimmunity and inflammation promise to get us much closer to a real understanding of how arthritis develops. And that could lead to ways of preventing it.

# 4 Effects of arthritis

Nearly everyone who has or thinks they may have arthritis is worried about becoming disabled – in the mind's eye is the dreaded wheelchair. Arthritis can cause severe physical disability, but this is uncommon and the effects are usually much less dramatic. Pain and frustration are among the commonest problems, but arthritis varies in the way in which it affects different people.

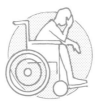

*In the mind's eye is the dreaded wheelchair.*

## Factors that determine effects of arthritis

The main things determining the variable effects of arthritis are:
- Which type of disease it is;
- How severe it is;
- How many and which joints are affected;
- How long the disease is active for;
- How the person reacts to having arthritis.

### Which disease?

Most types of arthritis rarely cause severe problems. Rheumatoid arthritis is most likely to lead to considerable handicap, but only about 10% of sufferers lose their independence.

### How severe?

The severity and activity of all the rheumatic diseases vary enormously in different people. Some long-standing, rheumatoid arthritis sufferers hardly even know they have a problem, others are painfully aware of their plight from the beginning.

## How many joints?

Disease of one joint is generally less of a problem than one that affects many parts of the body. Severe damage to one hip can be devastating, however, whereas mild arthritis of lots of joints may not cause too many difficulties. The outcome depends on which joints and how badly they are damaged, as well as the total number affected.

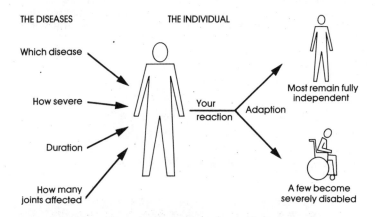

**Factors that determine effects of arthritis.**

## How long?

In some people arthritis remains active for only a few months or years; it then gets better either on its own or as a result of treatment. In others it goes on for many years. Generally speaking, the longer arthritis remains active the more likely it is to cause severe problems.

## How you react

There are plenty of reasons for believing that this is the most important factor in determining outcome. People who either give in too easily or cannot cope with all the problems their arthritis gives them may well have most troubles in the long run, even if the disease gets better. Those who react positively, learn how best to cope with the condition, respect but don't give in to it, and remain as cheerful and active as they can, will do well.

26

## The main effects of arthritis

The effects of arthritis can be split into three:
- The symptoms of joint disease, such as pain;
- The change in function of the limbs or spine – the wobbly knee that won't let you climb the stairs, for example;
- The overall handicap that a person is experiencing. Handicap depends on your needs and aspirations, your ability to cope with the condition, general health and many other factors in addition to the severity of the arthritis.

### Symptoms

*Pain*  Pain is a very personal thing – only you know how severe and how unpleasant it is. Some people feel dreadful pain even though there is little or no damage to the body; others seem to experience no pain in spite of extensive disease.

Pain is probably the most important symptom for most arthritis victims. Joint pain varies enormously in its quality, severity and characteristics. Sometimes it's an ache, sometimes a sharp, stabbing sensation. Some people experience other sorts of pain – always unpleasant and often unpredictable. It is often difficult to pinpoint the site of joint pain as it may be felt some distance away from the trouble causing it. A bad hip may cause pain in the knee, for example. Most chronic sufferers learn ways of coping with pain and treatment helps control it. But it is always there and, as yet, there is no way of getting rid of it completely. New ways are being explored, and research has detected some of the causes for its variability and idiosyncracies.

---

**The battle against pain is one of the big problems in arthritis, for everyone involved.**

---

*Stiffness*  Stiffness, or difficulty in getting joints to move properly, is another common problem in arthritis. It may be worse after a night's rest, or in the evening, or after sitting still for a while. Many people find they have to 'work their joints in' to get going.

*Feeling 'rotten'*   People with arthritis often say that they feel terribly tired and unwell. This is due to a combination of the hard work it takes to fight pain and stiffness and the activity of the arthritis in the body. It can be very disabling and is often not appreciated by anyone except the victim. This makes it that much more difficult to cope with.

*Depression*   Try not to let arthritis 'get you down'. It's hardly surprising that it often does. Again, this can be partly the effect of inflammation and active arthritis in the body, as well as the more obvious reason.

*Frustration*   For some people this is by far the biggest problem. If arthritis seems to be getting in the way of things, the anger and frustration that result can be very destructive. If you have this problem you need more help in coming to terms with it – talking about it, sharing, thinking about helping others even worse off than you are and just getting to know more about your disease can help.

### Loss of joint function

Arthritis can damage the joint so that normal movement and usage is affected in several ways.

*Locked joints*   Joints sometimes 'lock', or get stuck in one position for a minute or two. This can be very painful, and is caused by something catching inside. It usually lasts for only a short time. Other people find that their joints seem to 'give way'. This is usually caused by weakness of the muscles around the joint, although loss of stability of the joint itself can also occur. Typically a knee seems to buckle under as you try to get up or climb a step. Fortunately, joints never give way completely, although they can dislocate.

*Loss of movement*   A commoner problem is loss of movement of a joint. If a knee or hip won't move properly, walking and stair climbing are a problem. If it's the shoulders or elbows, it may mean you can't comb your hair or put on a bra, for example. Hand function is sometimes badly affected by stiff joints. Often problems arise from a combination of different joint problems in an arm or leg.

## The handicap caused by arthritis

Handicap can be defined as the total effect of the arthritis on your life. It is the result of a combination of symptoms, changes in joint function, your reaction and adaptation to the problem, and your particular needs and life style.

An example might help. If an elderly person gets arthritis that affects just the right knee, causing some pain and a bit of stiffness, it might not pose much of a problem. But the same arthritis in a young man who is embarking on a career as a professional footballer could be a disaster. The resulting handicap would be much greater for the young man than it would be for the pensioner. Or would it? Perhaps the young man would realise that it was silly to continue with a sporting career and turn to accountancy without any great regrets. Perhaps the pensioner would find the knee discomfort the last straw, and let it get him down to such an extent that it became a disproportionately big problem; we all see old people fall into that trap.

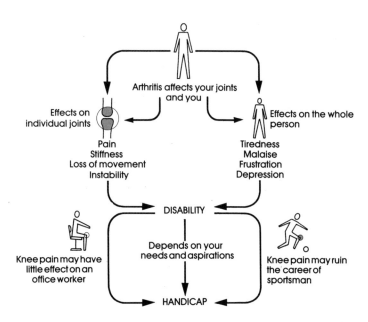

**Arthritis, disability and handicap.**

### It's up to you

So the handicap is up to you in some ways. It is more than the pain, the frustration and the joints not working properly. It is how you let it run your life and what you let the arthritis do to you.

> **Don't let the arthritis get on top and handicap you!**

# 5 Osteoarthritis

Osteoarthritis is easily the most common and important form of joint disease. It has had many other names, including 'degenerative joint disease' and 'osteoarthrosis', and it is often called 'OA' for short. The disease damages the surface of the joint so that it cannot function painlessly and properly. Osteoarthritis is not a single disease; it really describes joint failure, which can result from many different disorders and causes.

## Who gets osteoarthritis?

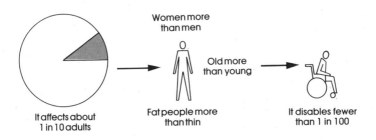

It affects about 1 in 10 adults — Women more than men — Old more than young — Fat people more than thin — It disables fewer than 1 in 100

Osteoarthritis can occur in any individual, male or female, throughout the animal kingdom. It is rare in man before the 30s or 40s, and symptoms commonly first appear in the 50s. Women are affected a little more often than men and some families are more prone to the condition than others. Any severe damage to a joint increases the chances of osteoarthritis developing at that site, and overweight people are more likely to get it than others.

Osteoarthritis is very variable, and often so mild that a sufferer never has to seek any medical help. Probably it affects around five million people in Britain – about one in every ten. Although it is often mild, some sufferers do have severe joint damage, pain and disability, and because of this osteoarthritis is the single biggest cause of disability in Britain today.

## What causes osteoarthritis?

In osteoarthritis a combination of factors is usually more important than any single cause. Ageing of joints is obviously important and so is being a woman. And our genetic make-up can make us more prone – in other words some of us are born with joints that are more likely to fail.

### Osteoarthritis is a battleground

After that, we can look on the causes of osteoarthritis as a battleground between mechanical factors that can damage the joints and the resilience of the body and its ability to repair any damage. Normal joints, used normally, will never get osteoarthritis, however long you live. Sportsmen and others who make special demands on their joints are no more likely to get it than anyone else unless they have severe injuries. Anything that causes a lot of disease or damage in a joint, however, does make it prone to osteoarthritis. So a professional footballer who has a succession of knee injuries and cartilage operations is more likely to get osteoarthritis of his knee than a tennis player or a cricketer.

### Primary and secondary osteoarthritis

Osteoarthritis can therefore be the result of another form of arthritis – it can occur, for example, after fractured bones, gout or rheumatoid arthritis (this is sometimes called secondary osteoarthritis). Conversely, if the cartilage and other tissues of the joint are a little weaker than normal, if the structure of the joint is a bit abnormal so that it is put under special stress, or if the repair process in the joints isn't as good as it should be, joints can develop the disorder without any previous damage or injury (this is known as primary osteoarthritis).

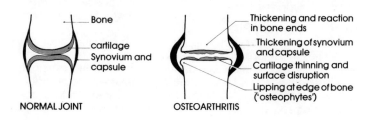

NORMAL JOINT — Bone / cartilage / Synovium and capsule

OSTEOARTHRITIS — Thickening and reaction in bone ends / Thickening of synovium and capsule / Cartilage thinning and surface disruption / Lipping at edge of bone ('osteophytes')

## How does it affect the joints?

The biggest changes occur in the cartilage surface of the joint and the bone immediately underneath. First, the surface of the cartilage becomes roughened. Later there is thinning and further breakdown of the cartilage, which may be almost completely worn away. The bone itself thickens and changes its shape a little. It also forms outgrowths – spurs – at the edges of the joint, called 'osteophytes'. These outgrowths are partly responsible for the gnarled appearance of the hands of some old people with the disorder. The lining membranes, the synovium and capsule, also thicken and become mildly inflamed, particularly in the more advanced stages. When the joint is severely damaged it may become mis-shapen and unstable, putting stresses on the ligaments and other tissues outside the joint and damaging them as well.

**Osteoarthritis affects only joints; it does not damage any other parts of the body and is not connected with other diseases.**

### Attempts at repair

Much of what is going on in a joint affected by osteoarthritis is part of the body's attempt to repair damage. The thickening of the bone and capsule is part of the healing response, and the cartilage itself, when examined minutely, shows plenty of evidence of attempted repair. Sometimes the joints do heal. They often stabilise after a certain degree of damage, and only a minority progress to severe changes. The joint is a battleground of forces tending to cause more damage against the body's defence and repair processes.

## Which joints are affected?

The joints most often damaged are the knee, the hip, and some of the joints in the hands and feet, including the bases of

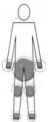

Osteoarthritis most often affects the knees, hips, ankles and hands.

the big toe (the bunion joint) and thumb, and the joints at the ends of the fingers. Some joints in the back are affected too. Osteoarthritis occurs less commonly at other sites. Some people have only one damaged joint, particularly if osteoarthritis follows a major injury, but usually a few joints are affected, the most frequent combination being knees or hips with hands and feet, with or without the spine.

## Symptoms and signs

Osteoarthritis is one of those conditions that usually starts slowly – it tends to creep up on you without an obvious, sudden beginning. Sometimes, however, affected joints get worse suddenly, often, for example, after a minor injury. The symptoms vary greatly and may be affected by changes in activity or the weather.

### Pain and stiffness

Pain is the main symptom. It varies from a mild ache to a deep, gnawing pain and is usually worse when the joints are being used and at the end of the day. Pain is often accompanied by stiffness. Mild joint stiffness first thing in the morning and more severe 'gelling' or sticking of the joints after a period of rest or inactivity are characteristic. Some people often find it very difficult to get their joints moving after sitting down for a while. Other symptoms that may be present include tenderness over the joints and cracking sensations or even locking of the joint on movement.

**Swelling**

Osteoarthritic joints don't swell up very much. There is often mild, firm swelling at the edges of damaged joints, and these areas may be tender. You may have knobbly swellings over the finger joints – these are called Heberden's or Bouchard's nodes after the doctors who first described them. A little fluid often forms in knee joints. The muscles around the joints may get thinner and weaker than normal and the joints generally creak a little when you move them. You cannot usually hear this creaking (called crepitus) but it can be felt by placing a hand over the moving joint. It sometimes occurs in normal joints, but tends to be more pronounced in osteoarthritis. You usually can't move the joint as much as before and pain tends to be at its worst as the joint is moved to the extremes of its range.

**Nodal osteoarthritis**

A special form of osteoarthritis sometimes occurs, especially in women around the time of the menopause. It affects the finger joints particularly, and behaves rather differently from other forms. It can start fairly abruptly, with more inflammation, heat and redness around the joints than usual. It generally settles after a few years leaving knobbly, stiff finger joints which usually function reasonably well without much pain. This form is called 'nodal' or 'generalised' osteoarthritis, and sometimes affects joints outside the hand.

## Complications

Osteoarthritis affects only the joints. Usually just a few are damaged and the sufferer is otherwise normal. There are no associated diseases apart from the links with overweight and raised blood pressure which occur in some sufferers. Osteo-arthritis is not a life-threatening or necessarily progressive illness and it often improves.

**Sudden worsening**

The only complication is a sudden worsening of an affected joint – this does happen sometimes, particularly in older people. There are two possible reasons. Sometimes a few calcium crystals form in the joint. If dislodged they can set up inflammation and make the joint worse (see p. 67). Alternatively, part of the surface of a damaged joint can suddenly collapse causing severe pain and stiffness. The joints don't dislocate or disintegrate, but they can deteriorate rapidly. Fortunately this occurs only in a very few sufferers.

## What tests are helpful?

The main investigation is an x-ray, which enables the doctor to see how abnormal the joint is. Damage to the cartilage causes a narrowing of the space between the bones, and the changes in the bone can also be seen, particularly the thickening (sclerosis) and the nodules (osteophytes).

### Blood tests, scans, etc

Other tests add little. Special ways of showing up the anatomy of a damaged joint are occasionally helpful, especially if any surgery is contemplated. These include joint scans, and special x-ray films taken after dye has been injected into the joints. It is sometimes useful to examine a drop of fluid (aspiration) from a joint to assess any inflammation and see if there are any crystals.

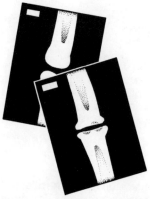

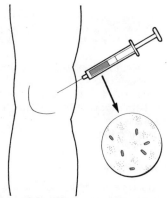

X-rays are the most important tests

Fluid withdrawn from a joint may show crystals when examined under a microscope

## How is osteoarthritis treated?

Unfortunately, there is no cure for osteoarthritis, but your symptoms can be eased considerably in a variety of ways.

### Reduce the stress on joints

The joint pain often comes from secondary stresses and strains put on the surrounding muscles, ligaments and tendons, or from pressure on or in the underlying bone. Much of this can be relieved by sensible reduction of the stress on the joint. Use of a walking stick decreases the pressure on a damaged hip or knee, for example, and a support may help badly damaged unstable joints. People who are overweight should diet to get their weight down and relieve the stress on their joints, but most relief of stress comes from building up good muscles around the joints, and physiotherapists can often help with this. Regular, gentle exercises that keep your muscles strong are very helpful. You should not rest too much but too much activity is also bad, so 'little and often' is probably the best approach. Intersperse periods of activity with periods of rest.

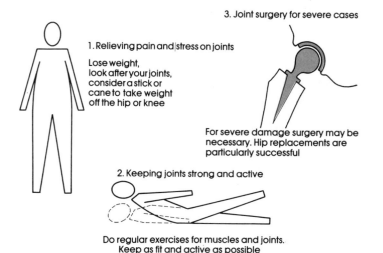

3. Joint surgery for severe cases

1. Relieving pain and/stress on joints

Lose weight, look after your joints, consider a stick or cane to take weight off the hip or knee

For severe damage surgery may be necessary. Hip replacements are particularly successful

2. Keeping joints strong and active

Do regular exercises for muscles and joints. Keep as fit and active as possible

## Mary

Mary is 68 and has had trouble with her knees for years. She has always been a bit on the plump side, just like her mother. Mary's fingers were also a bit painful some years ago, and they are lumpy at the ends, but they don't bother her much now.

It's her knees that are the problem. She can't remember quite when it started, it was probably about 10 years ago, and it slowly got worse without her really noticing any change. The knees, especially the right one, got more and more painful when she was walking to the shops or climbing the stairs. She also noticed that they got stuck after she sat down in the evenings. Mary has good days and bad days – when it's wet they often hurt more. She has some pills for the bad times; they seem to take the edge off the pain. Her doctor also sent her to the physiotherapist who taught her some exercises (which have certainly helped) and told her to lose some more weight.

Mary's knees have become knobbly and she is much more bow-legged than she used to be. The only good thing about her arthritis is that it does seem to have stopped getting worse. She even wonders if it might be a bit less of a nuisance than last year. Everyone says she must keep going . . . and she will.

### Drug treatments

Although drugs will not affect the progress of the disease, they help relieve pain. All that may be needed are pain killers such as paracetamol or aspirin used from time to time, and sometimes a course of an anti-inflammatory drug. If your osteoarthritis is severe, however, more constant use of drugs may be necessary to keep the pain down and allow you to function normally. Drugs that help joints to heal are being developed but they aren't available yet. You hear a lot about the side effects of drugs used for arthritis, but the latest drugs are reasonably safe when used sensibly, and you should certainly not try to 'put up with the pain' for fear of side effects (see p. 91).

### Surgery

Joint replacement surgery has revolutionised the treatment of severe osteoarthritis, but is necessary in only a few cases. Hip replacement operations are now commonplace, although it is worth remembering that the first successful ones were introduced only 25 years ago. Knee replacements are becoming more popular, and other artificial joints are being developed. Another operation is sometimes preferable, particularly for knee disease and in younger patients. This is called osteotomy and involves cutting through the bone near an affected joint and realigning it. Osteotomy relieves pain and pressure from the bone and stimulates healing of the joint.

### Other treatments

Other treatments that are sometimes useful include injecting joints and washing them out (p. 98). The occupational therapist can also advise people how to reduce stress on their joints and manage everyday tasks in spite of their limitations.

## What can you expect?

Things usually change slowly in osteoarthritis; it generally starts gradually, perhaps getting worse over a period of a year or two. A few people get better again and may have little or no trouble for the rest of their lives. In most people, however, there is a slow, variable period of worsening problems over a few years; then the osteoarthritis stabilises and the symptoms get a little easier. You will probably find it easier to adapt to the discomfort, limitations and frustration and manage to· live a reasonably normal sort of life. A few people, however, find that their osteoarthritis just goes on getting worse, or is complicated by a sudden deterioration. These are the people who may need joint surgery.

# 6 Rheumatoid arthritis

Rheumatoid arthritis is probably the rheumatic disease that people fear most. It can cause severe, crippling joint damage and a number of complications, but most sufferers manage well and keep pretty cheerful. The fear of the unknown can be much worse than the reality of the disease.

Rheumatoid arthritis affects only humans, and it may be relatively new; there seems little trace of it in Europe before AD 1800.

## Who gets rheumatoid arthritis?

Rheumatoid arthritis has been found in all parts of the world and in all races. It tends to be more severe, however, and may also be more common in Northern Europe. Women are affected about three times more often than men. It can start at any time of life, but most frequently begins in early adulthood, or around the time of the female menopause. Overall, in Britain, around one in every 200 women and one in every 600 men get the disorder. This means that there are around 250 000 sufferers, about a third of whom become severely disabled.

It is hard to predict who will get rheumatoid arthritis. If lots of people in your family have it, you have a greater than average chance, but you are still not severely at risk. There are no other clues; the disease seems to be no respecter of colour, class, creed or environment.

## What causes rheumatoid arthritis?

Rheumatoid arthritis is one of the conditions in which environmental factors seem to trigger disease in those who are born with a susceptibility to it.

### Genetic factors

More is known about the genetic background than the environment factors in rheumatoid arthritis. Several genes seem to be involved – some may control how bad the disease gets, whereas others (such as one called HLA D4) probably dictate your chances of getting it in the first place.

**Environmental factors**

The environmental factors are less well understood. A virus might act as the trigger in those with the right (or wrong!) genes. The fact that rheumatoid arthritis is now found everywhere tends to argue against some specific, local pollutant or dietary influence. It is possible that a number of different factors are involved and it also seems likely that some have more to do with the severity of rheumatoid arthritis, while others are important as trigger factors.

**Autoimmunity**

Rheumatoid arthritis is also one of several diseases in which 'autoimmune' phenomena occur. This means that the immune system, which normally defends us against infection, is reacting against some part of the body itself. It is possible that the problem in rheumatoid arthritis is that the genes make the immune response attack the joints.

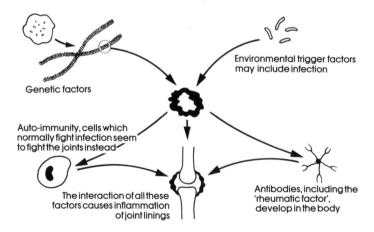

Genetic factors

Environmental trigger factors may include infection

Auto-immunity, cells which normally fight infection seem to fight the joints instead

The interaction of all these factors causes inflammation of joint linings

Antibodies, including the 'rheumatic factor', develop in the body

We still don't understand the causes of rheumatoid arthritis, but it seems that environmental trigger factors start the disease in a genetically susceptible person and an abnormal immune reaction then helps to keep the disease going.

## What happens in the joints?

The changes in the joints are easier to understand. The lining membrane, the synovium, becomes inflamed – swollen, red and hot because the blood vessels open up. Excess fluid and cells leak out of the inflamed membrane so that the whole joint becomes swollen and painful.

As the disease progresses, the inflamed membrane gradually begins to eat into the cartilage and the bone to form 'erosions'. This leads to the damage and deformity of advanced rheumatoid arthritis.

### Inflammation in tendons and bursae

The same inflammation can occur in the linings of tendons and bursae, and they can be damaged as well. If tendons are inflamed, movement is painful and difficult and the tendons occasionally snap. Some people develop 'nodules', which are patches of the same sort of inflammation occurring on tendons or just under the skin. The same process occasionally affects other parts of the body, including the lining of the heart or lungs, the eye, nerves, blood vessels in the skin and the kidneys. Rheumatoid arthritis is a generalised disease in which the inflammation is most likely to be in joints, but can occur in lots of other places too.

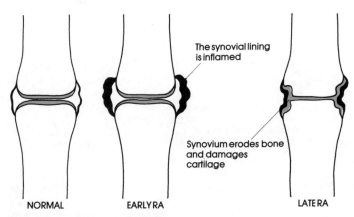

The synovial lining is inflamed

Synovium erodes bone and damages cartilage

NORMAL      EARLY RA      LATE RA

**How rheumatoid arthritis affects joints.**

## Why does inflammation last for so long?

One of the mysteries is the way in which this joint inflammation goes on for so long and causes so much damage. Inflammation occurs in lots of diseases, but it is often helpful, limiting the area of damage and getting the healing reaction started. Inflammation usually stops naturally when the job is done. But in rheumatoid arthritis it keeps on for no obvious reason and seems to *cause* the damage to the joints rather than helping. The abnormal immune defence mentioned in the preceding section is part of the answer. Much current research is aimed at trying to understand and control the abnormal immune reaction and the persistent inflammation which are at the heart of the disease.

## Symptoms and signs

If any part of your body is inflamed two things happen. First, there is pain and swelling at the site of the inflammation and secondly, you feel tired and unwell. The main feature of rheumatoid arthritis is severe inflammation in many joints, and sometimes in other parts of the body as well. It is therefore a painful condition and one which makes you feel as if you have 'flu most of the time.

### The onset

Rheumatoid arthritis occasionally starts suddenly – overnight for example. But more often it creeps up on people over the course of a few weeks or months. The joints first affected are generally in the hands and feet – more central joints are usually affected later. The joints become stiff and painful to move; there may be visible swelling, and the surrounding muscles become weaker. Joint stiffness first thing in the morning is usually quite severe and it may take hours for you to loosen up. The inflammation also makes you feel tired, irritable and unwell. You may have mild sweats at night, and are likely to lose weight. It may take a little while before you or your doctor realise that this is more than the general tiredness and aching of joints that anyone can get when stressed or exhausted. If swelling becomes obvious, however, and joint movement is affected the diagnosis becomes easier.

## The active phase

Rheumatoid arthritis tends to be most active in the first few years. After that it can go away completely, although it usually settles into a less vicious, but chronic phase.

The number and types of joint affected vary. The hands, wrists, feet and knees are almost always involved, but hips, shoulders, elbows, jaw and the neck may be affected too. The disease generally spares the back, but may be especially severe in any individual joint. Rheumatoid arthritis also waxes and wanes and most sufferers have 'flare-ups'. These sometimes follow too much activity but as often as not there is no apparent reason. The flare-ups may last days, weeks or even months before subsiding and the pain, stiffness, tiredness and ill health are all much worse during this time.

Most people with active disease sleep fitfully, wake up feeling very stiff and rotten, and have to loosen up their joints slowly. After an hour or so things improve a little and the best part of the day follows. You may need a rest mid-day, and start to get tired and to stiffen up again in the afternoon or early evening. You feel unwell and have to do many things slowly. The joints are often swollen, hot and very tender.

## Chronic rheumatoid arthritis

After an unpredictable time, usually several years, the disease begins to quieten down. During the active phase a variable degree of joint damage is being done by the inflamed synovium. This causes deformity, loss of joint stability, weakness of joints and reduced ranges of movement, and these problems will persist. The changes are often most obvious in the hands. But deformed hands may function quite well, and are often much less painful in chronic rheumatoid arthritis than they were in the active phase when they looked more presentable. In contrast, damage to larger joints, like the hips or knees, can cause devastating functional problems with considerable handicap as well as pain.

---

**People with chronic rheumatoid arthritis often feel better than they did, and their deformed hands and feet may not bother them too much, but some are on sticks or worse because of the amount of damage done to the main joints of the body.**

---

## Complications

Four types of complication occur:
- Local changes at the site of inflamed joints or nodules;
- Rheumatoid inflammation in other organs;
- The physical and psychological consequences of long-standing disease;
- Complications of treatment.

### Local complications

Swelling and inflammation can cause fluid to push its way out of the joint into the surrounding tissues to form a cyst. Inflammation can cause tendons to snap and can also put pressure on nerves – at the wrist, elbow and ankle, for example. Rarely, where the neck is affected, there is pressure on spinal nerves or the spinal cord, which can be quite serious. Local nodules sometimes have pressure effects as well, occasionally causing damage inside the body, but more commonly leading to ulceration of the overlying skin.

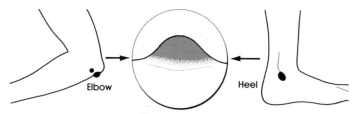

Elbow                                    Heel

Under the microscope you can see that nodules are chronic inflammatory swellings.

### Rheumatoid inflammation elsewhere

Rheumatoid arthritis causes inflammation of the linings of the joints (the synovium). The same inflammation and nodules can affect the lining of the lung, heart and eye. The blood vessels themselves may become inflamed and this can result in damaged nerves, severe ulceration of the skin, and occasionally gangrene. Anaemia is common, and reflects the amount of inflammation going on in the joints. Scarring of the lungs can occur and thinning of the bones as well as the skin is not uncommon.

### Physical and psychological damage

Constant pain and disability have their own consequences, often including anxiety, depression, and a reduced tolerance of further pain or suffering (see p. 27). Not surprisingly, some people are overwhelmed by bad rheumatoid arthritis and become withdrawn, demoralised and even more inactive than is necessary. Inactivity makes bone thinning and muscle wasting worse and can cause skin damage. Infections are more likely and the joints themselves can seize up totally. It is very important therefore to keep going and keep on top of the disease.

### Complications of treatment

As explained below, most people get great benefit from treatment. But the treatment is far from perfect and can cause its own problems, such as stomach troubles including peptic ulceration, caused by arthritis drugs. Other rare problems include rashes, blood disorders and kidney damage.

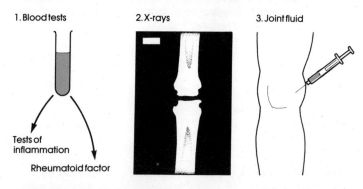

1. Blood tests    2. X-rays    3. Joint fluid

Tests of inflammation

Rheumatoid factor

## What tests are helpful?

If you have rheumatoid arthritis is is likely that your doctor will want to do regular blood tests and x-rays, but he may wish to do other, more specialised tests as well. The purposes are:
- To confirm the diagnosis early on in the disease;
- To assess the activity of the disease, its progression and the effects of any complications;
- To help assess the effects of any treatments and judge whether they are likely to be of continuing benefit.

## Diagnosis

Diagnosis can be assisted by blood tests.

The ESR (erythrocyte sedimentation rate) is one of a number of blood tests that give doctors an idea of the presence and amount of inflammation going on. The blood may be tested for a substance called rheumatoid factor, which is detectable in about 5% of the normal population, but occurs in about 80% of rheumatoid arthritis sufferers, often in quite a large quantity.

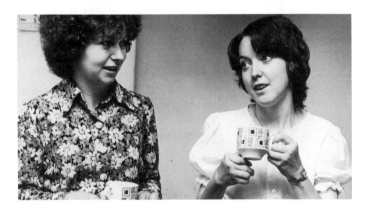

The x-rays may show the characteristic erosions of bone at the edge of affected joints, although it is usually some months or years before they can be seen. If there is fluid on a joint, such as the knee, examination of this sometimes helps. None of these tests is absolute confirmation of the diagnosis, but they help sort out the likely type of arthritis early on.

## Disease activity

This is assessed by the same types of blood test (ESR, rheumatoid factor, and others), assisted by x-rays and sometimes synovial fluid tests. The presence of *complications* may be detected only by special assessments of the lungs, heart or kidneys, for example. The *progression* of the arthritis is judged by examinations and by any changes that occur on the x-rays. *Treatment* may need to be monitored by regular blood and urine tests to make sure that no damage is being done, so that the drugs can be stopped before any permanent harm occurs.

### Assessing treatment

As the disease is developing and responding to different forms of treatment, some of the blood tests in particular may show changes (for good or bad) before there is any effect on the joints or how the sufferer is feeling. Doctors are developing better ways of assessing disease activity and treatment, and looking for the best tests to predict the eventual outcome and the effect of treatment so that the best treatment can be given early on. Some quite different forms of test can help in this, including questionnaires about joint function and a variety of measurements of pain, movement and the psychological effects such as depression.

## How is rheumatoid arthritis treated?

The treatment of rheumatoid arthritis needs to be 'holistic' – it needs to consider all aspects of the patient and his or her environment.

### Understanding helps

Education and understanding help. Rheumatoid arthritis affects family and friends as well as the sufferer, and everyone needs to know something about it. Discussions with doctors and therapists as well as pamphlets and books like this one should help. Getting rheumatoid arthritis has been likened to a bereavement. You tend to go through the same stages of shock, anger, depression and acceptance. Losing some of your independence can be like losing a loved one, and it can be just as hard to take. You need help to get to the point of acceptance – and the disease seems to be kinder to people when they come to terms with it.

### Keep moving

It is very important to respect the condition and the inflammation going on in the joints, but equally vital to keep them moving, maintain as much activity as possible, and keep your muscles strong. The balance between rest and exercise can be difficult to get right, and is different for each person. In general, rest helps inflammation and flare-ups, and activity helps keep joints supple and strong. 'Little and often' is a good rule for

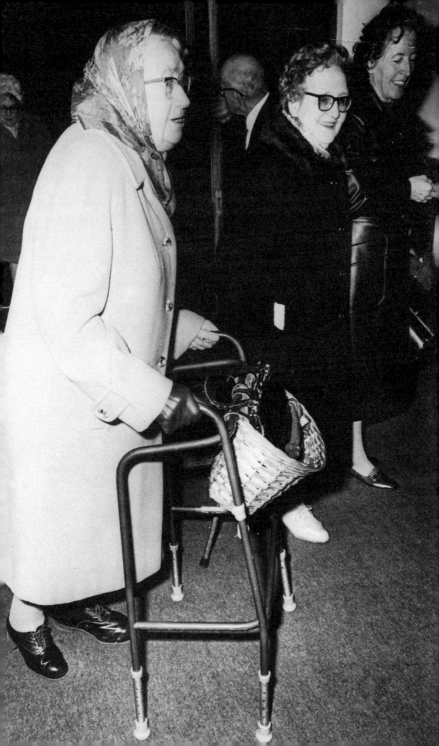

exercise, and doing a little too much is generally better than doing too little. The therapists can help advise about joint protection and appropriate exercises.

## Drug treatments

There are two main types of drug treatment – drugs that relieve symptoms and those that treat the disease process. Anti-inflammatory drugs are the mainstay of symptom treatment. They are relatively simple and safe, and they give most sufferers a lot of relief from pain and stiffness. Anti-inflammatory drugs don't, however, stop the disease or affect its outcome but a number of other drugs are now available to reduce disease activity and slow down joint damage; they can also make people feel much better in themselves. Drugs of this type include gold injections, a tablet form of gold salt, antimalarial drugs like hydroxychloroquine, drugs used in the treatment of cancer and those that suppress the body's immune response, a substance chemically similar to penicillin, called d-penicillamine, and· an aspirin derivative called sulphasalazine. All these drugs take several weeks or months to work and can cause side effects. The response to them varies and is unpredictable, but is often very good. It is not known how they work, but the continuing improvements in their usage is having an excellent overall effect on disease control and outcome.

## Other approaches

Many other 'chemical' approaches to treatment are used, including diets, herbal remedies, homoeopathy, substances rubbed into joints, and a variety of odd animal, plant or mineral extracts. Some of these do occasionally help, but when formal tests have been done on groups of rheumatoid arthritis sufferers they come out as much less effective than the drugs mentioned above (see p. 107)

## Severe disease

In severe or advanced disease, splints, walking and other aids, and a variety of appliances can improve independence immensely and make life much easier. The therapists (p. 98) can help at all stages. Injections into joints can give temporary relief to inflamed joints, and sometimes more lasting benefit. Surgery (p. 102) can also play an important part in severe rheumatoid arthritis.

## Outcome

Anyone who has read this chapter straight through could be thoroughly depressed by this point! Don't be – it is not all bad: rheumatoid arthritis is very variable and most people don't get any of the serious complications and remain independent.

**Be positive**

Out of every 100 people who get rheumatoid arthritis, about a third will get considerable disability and handicap, 5 or 10 will get completely better, and the remaining 60 or so will have continuing pain and problems, but will be able to keep going. Treatment does help and is getting better. A positive attitude is one of the best predictors of a good outcome – start now!

## Conclusion

Rheumatoid arthritis is the most serious of the common forms of arthritis. This chapter can provide only an introduction to it but many other chapters in this book expand on various issues of relevance to rheumatoid arthritis sufferers, and the people and organisations quoted should be able to provide more information and help.

### Brenda

Brenda is 56 and has had rheumatoid arthritis for 19 years. It is part of her. It started gradually – to begin with she just felt rotten and achy, and things were a struggle in the morning. Then her hands and feet became stiff and painful, and one of her knees began to swell. The mornings became increasingly difficult; it was a real struggle to get going and get everyone breakfast. She was getting tearful and depressed. So Jack took her to the doctor. He took some blood tests and gave her some tablets which helped a bit. When she saw him again he looked worried. He told her she had arthritis and had better see a specialist. By the time the specialist confirmed the diagnosis and told them more about the disease, the effects were becoming more obvious. Brenda's fingers were swollen and stiff; she was having trouble with lots of everyday jobs and was always losing her temper with the family.

The first few years were the worst. Brenda got worse, physically and mentally, and had a couple of spells in hospital. Jack and the children were confused and unhappy. It seemed as if everything was being taken away from the family and that everything had to revolve round Mum's arthritis. But slowly things got better. The people at the hospital and some of their friends helped. The family began to adjust and find that most things were possible after all. After a difficult few years it seems to have brought them all together; they are now a close, happy family again.

Brenda is quite disabled; she has severe rheumatoid arthritis. She gets around the house slowly, with the help of sticks, but can't manage the stairs or get out much without Jack's help. Her hands are very deformed, she needs help dressing and can't do much in the kitchen. Several changes have been made in parts of the house to help Brenda, and she has a number of aids so that she can manage when alone. She still goes to the hospital regularly, and is on tablets which still help.

But Brenda is cheerful in spite of the constant pain and disability. She has a circle of good friends who come to see her and take her out when Jack's at work. She is a member of a couple of local clubs, and contributes to a lot of charity work. She says she has stopped being angry or depressed now.

# 7 Ankylosing spondylitis and related disorders

Ankylosing spondylitis is a form of arthritis in which the joints in the back become inflamed and then stiffen up. It is one of a family of related diseases that can cause inflammation in the skin, eyes and other parts of the body, as well as in the spine and limb joints. Other conditions in this group include reactive arthritis and Reiter's disease, psoriatic arthritis and colitic arthritis. (The medical term for the whole group is the 'seronegative spondarthropathies'!)

## Some explanation

The names used may need explanation. 'Spondylitis' means inflammation of the spine, and 'ankylosing' just means stiffening or fixation of joints. The name describes the result of the disease. 'Reactive arthritis' is a condition in which joints become inflamed after an infection in some other part of the body, usually the gut or genito-urinary tract. The arthritis is a short-lasting, abnormal 'reaction' to infection. Reiter's disease (named after a Hans Reiter) is one form of reactive arthritis. 'Psoriatic' arthritis is a term used to cover a number of forms of arthritis that can occur in people with the skin disease psoriasis. Similarly, 'colitic' arthritis simply means arthritis related to having the bowel disorder colitis.

All of these diseases can affect the spine and limb joints in a similar way. They share other features and all of them are more common in people with a specific genetic make-up. There are, however, also lots of differences between each disease in this group, so they are described separately.

## Ankylosing spondylitis

This condition usually affects young, adult men but women can get it as well. Ankylosing spondylitis tends to run in families, although lots of people with the disorder have no affected relatives and vice-versa.

### Genetic marker

Ankylosing spondylitis is strongly associated with a gene called HLA B27 (B27 for short). Between 5% and 10% of the normal population have B27, but over 90% of those with ankylosing spondylitis have it. Without B27 (which is inherited from one parent) you are unlikely to get the disease; if you have B27 you still have only about a 1 in 20 risk of getting it.

Although ankylosing spondylitis is a common disease, its incidence is difficult to work out. Many people have very mild disease and don't bother visiting the doctor. Noticeable disease probably occurs in about one in 1000 people, with men affected at least five times as often as women.

### What causes ankylosing spondylitis?

The fact that about one in 20 of those with B27 get ankylosing spondylitis suggests that some environmental trigger sets the disease going in those people genetically at risk. The environmental factor is unknown, however, and few clues have been found to explain the cause or why it starts when it does.

### What happens in the joints?

In ankylosing spondylitis and the other related diseases the symptoms and stiffness are caused by inflammation.

But it is quite a different sort of inflammatory reaction to the one that occurs in rheumatoid arthritis. There may be a mild reaction in the lining of joints, but the main feature is a chronic, inflammatory reaction at the edge of the joints, where tendons and ligaments are attached to bone. The other distinctive aspect is that this reaction tends to form scar tissue, which eventually turns into bone. It is this that causes the stiffness of the spine. As time goes by the scar tissue and bone may bridge the gap between two vertebrae, so that part of the back becomes completely rigid.

NORMAL

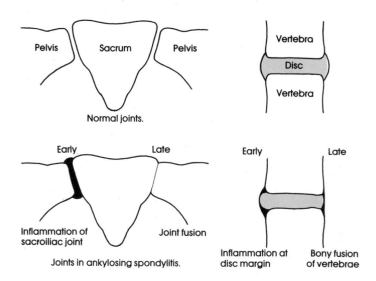

Normal joints.

Inflammation of sacroiliac joint | Joint fusion

Joints in ankylosing spondylitis.

Inflammation at disc margin | Bony fusion of vertebrae

A similar reaction can occur at the edges of joints outside the spine, particularly those around the pelvis and in the legs. Fortunately, however, this rarely leads to these joints becoming fused together.

### Symptoms and signs

Ankylosing spondylitis tends to start at the bottom of the back (in the sacroiliac joints) and travels up the spine over a time span of a few years. In a few sufferers, other joints such as shoulders, hips and knees are also affected. Many get episodes of inflammation at tendon insertions in various parts of the body.

Pain at the base of the spine and buttocks, sometimes travelling down the leg, is the commonest symptom. The pain is associated with spinal stiffness first thing in the morning and is often relieved by exercise. This helps distinguish it from other types of back pain. If ankylosing spondylitis starts in boys, it may begin with pain and swelling in a knee or ankle, rather than back problems.

Most people continue to have pain and early morning back stiffness for a number of years. It tends to travel up the spine so that symptoms become more extensive over the years. Exercise helps, but there is a gradual tendency for the back to become stiffer so that bending and stretching are difficult. The neck may be affected, and in more severe cases the hips get stiff and painful as well, which makes the loss of spine movement much more of a problem. Occasionally other joints are affected – episodes of pain around the heels, feet, pelvis and chest wall are common, especially early on.

The inflammation tends to subside after some years and the disease is quite likely to burn itself out around the age of 50 or so. As with most arthritic diseases, however, both the severity and the duration vary enormously. Many people have it so mildly that it is either no problem or a minor inconvenience; a few get severe disease and develop rigid, bent spines and stuck hips.

### Complications

The main complication is eye inflammation, which occurs in about 25% of people with ankylosing spondylitis. The membranes at the front of the eye become red and painful. This settles down within a few days if treated correctly and rarely damages the eye, but it is important to get prompt medical attention if it happens.

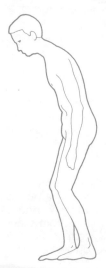

Ankylosing spondylitis produces a stooped posture unless treatment is given to prevent this.

Apart from the chance of joints outside the spine being affected, other complications are rare. Ankylosing spondylitis occasionally affects the aortic valve in the heart or causes scarring of the upper part of the lung. If the spinal disease is very bad so that the back is severely bent there may be additional complications including small fractures and pressures on nerves, but this is very uncommon.

## What tests are helpful?

The diagnosis of ankylosing spondylitis may be difficult in its early phase. Lots of people get back pain, and neither medical examination nor tests may show much for a year or so. Blood tests such as the erythrocyte sedimentation rate can be helpful in detecting inflammation. Once the disease has been present for a few years x-rays of the sacroiliac joints and lumbar spine leave no doubt as to the diagnosis. X-rays can also help to assess how the disease is progressing.

## Treatment

There is no cure for ankylosing spondylitis but the symptoms can be kept under control and severe stiffness or deformity of the spine can be prevented. The main treatment is *exercise*, which relieves pain as well as preventing deformity. Anyone with ankylosing spondylitis should do special exercises for their spine every day. Lying flat, face down, for a little while each day will stop you getting bent over, and paying attention to good posture at work or in the home will also help. Help from a physiotherapist is useful in severe cases, but mostly it is up to you to keep your exercise programme going at home.

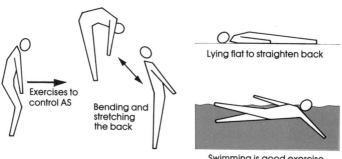

Exercises to control AS

Bending and stretching the back

Lying flat to straighten back

Swimming is good exercise

Anti-inflammatory drugs may also relieve pain and stiffness – a tablet or two last thing at night can be very helpful for stiffness first thing in the morning.

Other measures, such as different drugs, x-ray treatment (largely a thing of the past), and operations are rarely used. Hip replacements can be necessary for those with severe hip damage, and just occasionally the spine gets bad enough to need surgery.

### Outcome

Most people with ankylosing spondylitis do well. Daily exercises, with or without tablets, keep them reasonably symptom-free, fit, active and supple. Some spinal stiffening and discomfort is usual, but it is generally mild enough to make relatively little impact on your life. Most people with ankylosing spondylitis are able to work and many continue with sport. The condition often burns out in later life. Only a few severely affected people end up needing hip surgery, get incapacitating stiffness in the back and neck, or have serious, recurrent eye problems.

## Reactive arthritis and Reiter's syndrome

In 1916, Hans Reiter described a group of soldiers with inflamed eyes (conjunctivitis) and arthritis after an epidemic of dysentery. The term 'Reiter's syndrome' was then used to describe conjunctivitis and arthritis after urogenital or bowel infections. Doctors subsequently realised that inflammation of the eyes, skin, urogenital tract, inside of the mouth, and joints could occur in a variety of combinations after bowel, urinary or genital infections. The general term 'reactive arthritis' covers the whole spectrum of combinations that can occur.

### Who and why?

Reactive arthritis affects young people, aged between 15 and 35, and is commoner in men than women. Most sufferers have the genetic marker B27. A variety of genital and bowel infections trigger the condition and it sometimes results from a minor sexually transmitted infection (non-specific urethritis). Exactly how it is caused is unknown.

## What happens?

Within a few days or weeks of the trigger infection, inflammation starts at one or more of the vulnerable sites. The commonest things are conjunctivitis, urethritis (causing a discharge from the penis and pain on passing water), mouth ulcers, a skin rash on the bottom of the feet, a rash on the penis (the cervix may be affected in women) and arthritis. Most other problems settle after a few weeks, but the arthritis is often more persistent and more of a problem.

The arthritis affects the legs more than the arms. Painful swelling of a knee, ankle or toes occurs and several joints may be affected. It usually lasts for a few months and then settles, although recurrences can occur. Joint damage is rare, but a few sufferers develop a long-standing, damaging leg arthritis or ankylosing spondylitis, or both.

## Treatment and outcome

The infection that acts as the trigger may need treating initially. The arthritis can be quite severe in the acute stage, and joints may need rest. Withdrawing some of the fluid around the joint and injections are sometimes required and anti-inflammatory drugs can be helpful. As the condition slowly settles activity can increase, and use of drugs decrease. Long-standing disease is rare but if it occurs other drugs and local treatments may be needed.

Reactive arthritis usually settles completely after a few weeks or months, and with luck, that is the end of it; no lasting damage or problems occur. Some people are unlucky, however, and get repeated recurrences of inflammation or develop ankylosing spondylitis or chronic joint disease, or both.

## Psoriasis and arthritis

Psoriasis is a relatively common skin disease, in which patches of inflammation occur in various parts of the body. They are red and scaly, but don't itch much. It can be very unsightly but varies a lot.

About one in every ten people with psoriasis gets arthritis as well. This can take a number of forms, and is very variable and unpredictable. It usually develops after the skin lesions, but the severity of one condition does not parallel that of the other.

A group of disorders with similarities

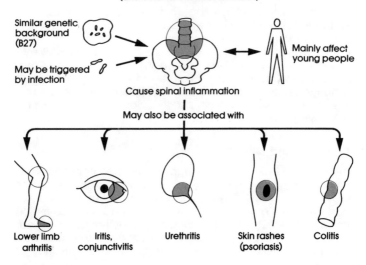

Ankylosing spondylitis
Psoriatic arthritis
Reactive arthritis
Colitic arthritis
(and other rare arthritic diseases)

Similar genetic background (B27)

May be triggered by infection

Cause spinal inflammation

Mainly affect young people

May also be associated with

Lower limb arthritis

Iritis, conjunctivitis

Urethritis

Skin rashes (psoriasis)

Colitis

### Types of psoriatic arthritis

The types of arthritis that can occur with psoriasis include:
- Ankylosing spondylitis;
- A generalised arthritis that is rather like rheumatoid arthritis. It is, however, less severe than rheumatoid arthritis and none of the complications outside joints that can happen in this disorder occur with psoriasis. Intermittent flare-ups in one or several joints are common and unpredictable;
- Arthritis of the joints at the ends of the fingers and in the toes. This can occur on its own, or with some other joint problems. Psoriasis can affect nails, and this form of arthritis tends to occur in fingers or toes with nail problems. It may just affect one end joint or a whole digit may swell up like a sausage (this can occur in reactive arthritis as well).
- Other forms of joint problem develop in people with psoriasis, including a very unusual destructive form of joint disease, but this is rare.

## Treatment

Relatively little is known about the cause but it seems likely that the sort of inflammation that occurs in the skin also affects the joints. Treating the skin doesn't affect the arthritis and the joints are treated according to the type of problem. In addition, there are a few drugs that can suppress both the skin and joint disease, including azathioprine and methotrexate. These drugs can have side effects, however, and are reserved for the uncommon, severe case of psoriatic arthritis.

## Colitis and arthritis

Colitis means inflammation of the bowel. The two main forms of this are ulcerative colitis and Crohn's disease, both of which are associated with arthritis in about 20% of patients.

Two main forms of arthritis can occur – ankylosing spondylitis and inflammation of the leg joints, rather like that seen in a reactive arthritis. The ankylosing spondylitis bears no relationship to the bowel disease, but the lower limb arthritis tends to occur when bowel inflammation is most active. Occasionally, other bowel diseases, such as rare disorders called Whipple's disease and coeliac disease, are associated with arthritis.

# 8 Gout, pseudogout and joint crystals

Gout is caused by deposits of uric acid crystals in joints. A build up of uric acid in the blood can lead to the crystals growing in various parts of the body, including the skin and kidney, but the joints are particularly vulnerable. Once the crystals are there they can shower out into the joint space, triggering an acute attack of inflammation; in other words an attack of gout. If large deposits remain in the joints for many years this can also cause permanent joint damage.

> **Nowadays gout is easy to treat and severe cases are rare.**

Calcium crystals can also grow in joints. They occasionally cause acute attacks of inflammation (pseudogout) and may be associated with long-term joint damage.

## Gout

Gout was described by Hippocrates, the Greek 'father of medicine', around 400 BC. Many famous people have suffered from it since, including past kings and prime ministers of England. Gouty men have a reputation for good living and port drinking – an idea which probably arose in the 17th and 18th centuries, when port was polluted with lead. Chronic lead poisoning can cause gout by damaging the kidney.

Gout is now easy to diagnose and fairly easy to treat. Although it is still quite a common form of arthritis, it is no longer the scourge it was and research has produced a good understanding of the disease and effective treatment.

## Who gets gout?

Gout affects men much more than women. It tends to run in families and usually starts in young adulthood or middle age. Sufferers are often of above average intelligence; they may also be overweight and have high blood pressure. It sometimes affects older women, especially those on diuretic drugs (water tablets) used to treat heart disorders and raised blood pressure. Gout is occasionally caused by a disease of the blood or kidneys, but this is rare and most sufferers are otherwise quite healthy.

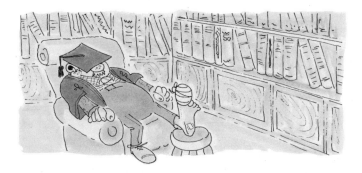

## What causes gout?

Gout can occur only if uric acid crystals grow in the joints. This happens in some people who have too much uric acid in their blood.

Uric acid is formed in the body when waste products are broken down to be reused. Most of us pass enough uric acid out in our urine to keep the levels in the blood low. People with gout, however, usually inherit a tendency to get rid of less uric acid than usual. Occasionally this is caused by eating or drinking large quantities of things that make uric acid in the body; or because the body is making too much uric acid on its own; or because drugs or damage to the kidney interfere with the body's ability to get rid of uric acid.

Not everyone with too much uric acid gets gout – the crystals have to grow in joints for that to happen. It seems that this is more likely to occur in some people than in others and in particular joints, such as the big toe. We still don't fully understand this. If there is a lot of uric acid in the blood it sometimes forms crystals in the kidney (to produce stones) or the skin (forming 'tophi') as well.

## What happens in the joints?

Uric acid crystals grow in the cartilage of the joint. They form slowly in bunches, producing a small lump of chalky material. If a large shower of crystals falls off into the joint space it causes inflammation in the joint lining. The cells in the synovium work like mad to get rid of the crystals and damp down the reaction. After a few days they usually win the battle and the attack of gout subsides. A few attacks cause little or no permanent damage, but repeated episodes or the build up of large deposits can eventually lead to wear and damage to the joint surface and underlying bone.

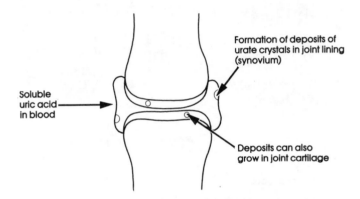

Formation of deposits of urate crystals in joint lining (synovium)

Soluble uric acid in blood

Deposits can also grow in joint cartilage

## Symptoms and signs in gout

Gout usually starts with an acute attack, most often at the base of the big toe. It may be triggered by a minor injury or illness – such as stubbing your toe or getting a cold – but it usually starts for no apparent reason. The toe starts to itch and over the period of only a few hours becomes red, swollen and excruciatingly painful. After a few days the pain and swelling slowly settle and eventually the joint returns to normal. Some variation on this pattern is not unusual. Other joints such as parts of the foot, ankle, hand or wrist, and occasionally the knee or elbow may be affected too. Sometimes more than one joint is affected at the same time, and occasionally a bursa or other area under the skin is more inflamed than a joint. The duration of an attack varies, but modern treatment can usually cope with the worst of the pain quite quickly.

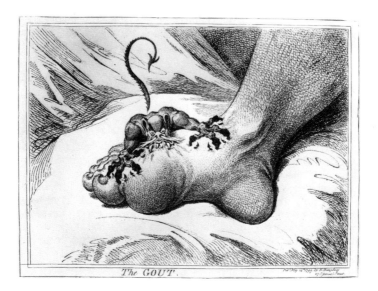

*Gout is excruciatingly painful.*

### Treatment is important

Many gouty men will have only one or two attacks a year, even if they don't seek treatment. But untreated gout tends to turn slowly into a more chronic phase – attacks may become more frequent, although less severe, and as time goes on the affected joints may become damaged, causing more constant pain. Deposits of crystals may form over the joints or in the ear. These are the tophi of gout, fortunately not often seen, because these features of chronic gout can be prevented by treatment.

### Complications and associated problems

Untreated gout can lead to widespread joint damage and tophi. The joints are then like those with severe osteoarthritis. Long-standing gout can lead to kidney stones and kidney damage as well. These complications are rare and unnecessary.

People with gout are often overweight and may have a high blood pressure, which if left untreated can lead to disease of the blood vessels such as a heart attack or stroke. These risks may be further increased by high blood levels of some fats;

and again this is not uncommon in gouty sufferers – but the problem is preventable by appropriate treatment. Keep your weight down, eat a sensible diet, and have regular blood pressure checks.

### What tests are helpful?

A blood test will show if there is too much uric acid in the body and urine tests may be necessary to find out if too little is being excreted by the kidney, rather than too much being made in the body. X-rays do not help diagnose acute gout, as the deposits do not show up, but evidence of joint damage can be seen if the gout is long-standing. The best test is to extract a little of the fluid from the joint and look at it under a microscope. The crystals of uric acid can then be identified. Your doctor may also want to check your blood pressure, kidney function, and the level of blood lipids (fats) because of the associated problems and complications mentioned above.

### How is gout treated?

There are three aspects to treatment:
- Quick relief of pain in an attack;
- Prevention of long-standing gout;
- Avoiding the risk of a heart attack or stroke.

Acute attacks are easy to treat. Any of the many different anti-inflammatory drugs (p. 93) will help, but don't use aspirin. The ancient remedy, colchicine, is still used sometimes, but other measures, such as injecting the affected joints or giving steroid drugs, are hardly ever necessary.

---

**Aspirin can increase the level of uric acid in the body and shouldn't be used to relieve the pain of gout.**

---

### Prevention

Preventing chronic gout is also fairly simple. Simply losing a little weight will help some patients reduce the amount of uric acid in the blood sufficiently. In others the levels are only slightly raised and nothing needs to be done. But many gouty patients do need treatment to prevent recurrent attacks and complications. Two sorts of drug can do this – one (allopurinol) prevents too much uric acid forming in the body; the others (there are several and probenicid is one) help the kidney to increase the amount of uric acid excreted. When either of these drugs is started the gout may temporarily get worse before it gets better. It is often necessary to take a low dose of an anti-inflammatory drug or colchicine as well for the first few weeks. Once established, a single daily dose is both very safe and effective in preventing any further gout problems.

### Avoiding other risks

The slightly increased risk of blood vessel problems present in some gouty men can also be treated. They should not be overweight, and high blood pressure should be controlled, as should excess fats in the blood. Like the rest of us, gout sufferers should keep fit and avoid cigarettes.

### Outcome

The outcome is excellent. Most sufferers live normal, healthy lives; get no appreciable joint damage; suffer no complications; and have a normal life-span. One or two tablets a day may be necessary to achieve this – a small price to pay.

## Calcium crystals: pseudogout and related diseases

A variety of calcium phosphate crystals can grow in the cartilage of joints. This becomes more common as people get older – a little will probably develop in all of us if we live long enough. Usually it does no harm, but just like a gouty deposit, some of the crystals can get dislodged – perhaps by an injury. This can set up an acute attack of inflammation a little like an acute attack of gout. It is not uncommon in elderly people and usually occurs in the knee joint. This type of attack is called 'pseudogout'; it is less painful than gout and slowly settles on its own. Attacks can be treated by anti-inflammatory drugs, or by drawing off the crystal-containing fluid from the swollen knee joint.

### Crystals and arthritis

In some elderly people, the growth of crystals in the joint cartilage contributes to the development of osteoarthritis. Unusual, severe forms of osteoarthritis can develop because of an- interaction of crystal deposits with an already damaged joint. These disorders have been given a number of names including 'pyrophosphate arthropathy'. Various different crystal types and several different types of joint damage have been described. Unfortunately there is no special treatment for this, and as yet there is no known way of getting rid of these crystals or stopping their formation. Research is being done, however, and we may soon have effective treatment of the sort used in gout.

## Andrew

Andrew is 49. His uncle suffered from gout, but he had forgotten all about that until it happened to him. It started soon after his 40th birthday. He woke up one night with a painful, itchy toe. By the middle of the next day he was in dreadful pain and thought his toe was going to burst. It was hot, red and swollen. He knew at once that it was gout and so did the emergency doctor, who gave him some tablets which helped the pain. He couldn't stand that day, and it was several days before he could walk normally, but after a week he was back to normal. He stopped the tablets, went back to work and forgot about it. After the third attack his wife Anne said he had to do something about it. She had been on about his weight and his beer drinking as well. Andrew went to his GP who did some blood tests, checked his blood pressure, and told him he had better lose some weight and stop drinking so much. He sounded just like Anne! The doctor also gave him a booklet which helped explain gout as well as some tablets for the blood pressure. Andrew goes to the surgery regularly now, he is two stones lighter, a lot fitter, and his blood pressure is fine as long as he keeps taking his tablets. His friends tease him about the gout, but aren't so happy to find that his golf has improved! Andrew keeps some tablets with him for the occasional attack of gout, but these are rare and he and his doctor have agreed that there is no need to take anything regularly. Anne keeps telling him that it is just as well that he got the gout or he might have had a heart attack like Uncle Paul.

# 9 Some uncommon forms of arthritis

As there are some 200 different forms of arthritis, a book like this cannot describe them all. Most of the commoner types have been mentioned already, but there are others that occur sometimes and should perhaps be mentioned. These include joint infections, diseases of the tissues that hold our bones and joints together, tumours, a miscellaneous group of odd rheumatic disorders, and a strange group generally known as 'connective tissue diseases'.

## Connective tissue diseases

This is a group of uncommon diseases that affect many parts of the body and share a number of common features. The group includes:
- Systemic lupus erythematosis;
- Scleroderma (systemic sclerosis);
- Mixed connective tissue disease;
- Sicca syndrome (Sjorgren's);
- Polymyositis;
- Dermatomyositis;
- Polyarteritis nodosa.

Most of these diseases occur mainly in young women. Although their cause is unknown, most are associated with quite severe disturbances of the immune system, and auto-immune reactions. In other words, much of the problem seems to arise from the immune defence system attacking various parts of your own body. Inflammation is the main result and it can occur in many organs, including joints. A variety of treatment is used to suppress both the immune disturbance and the inflammation, but there are no cures – these diseases remain something of a mystery in spite of a lot of research.

### Systemic lupus erythematosis

This is the commonest of these diseases. Young women are affected, and it is more frequent in some races than others (in

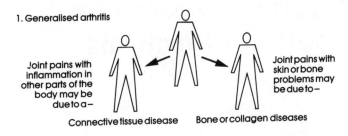

1. Generalised arthritis

Joint pains with inflammation in other parts of the body may be due to a –

Connective tissue disease

Joint pains with skin or bone problems may be due to –

Bone or collagen diseases

2. Localised arthritis

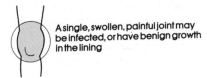

A single, swollen, painful joint may be infected, or have benign growth in the lining

**Rare forms of arthritis.**

the Chinese and Black Americans, for example). Systemic lupus erythematosis is a 'multisystem' disorder that causes skin rashes, arthritis, general tiredness and depression, and a host of other problems. In Britain, it is usually a fairly mild disease, although serious complications can occur in the kidney and elsewhere. It is one of those conditions that has flare-ups, and it can be worsened by exposure to sun and drugs, among other things.

The body produces antibodies that attack deoxyribonucleic acid (the acid that carries all our genetic information) in systemic lupus erythematosis; they can be measured in the blood, helping doctors make the diagnosis. There is no cure, but serious disease and flare-ups can be treated well with steroids and immunosuppressive drugs, and hydroxychloroquine tablets are often helpful. Rest helps active disease.

### Scleroderma (systemic sclerosis)

This also affects young women. It usually starts with Raynaud's phenomenon (see below), followed by the gradual development of thickening and tightening of the skin over the hands. It causes extra scar tissue to form in the skin and elsewhere for no apparent reason. This results in tight, thick skin, scarring in the oesophagus that can make swallowing difficult, and sometimes scars in the lung, kidney and elsewhere. Although it varies in severity and can cause serious problems, most cases are not too bad, and scleroderma often stops progressing after a few years. There is no effective treatment.

## Mixed connective tissue disease

This extraordinary name describes a rare condition that combines various features of systemic lupus erythematosis and scleroderma. The disease has a reasonably favourable outlook but severe Raynaud's phenomenon (see below) is one of the biggest problems.

## Sicca syndrome

In this condition the glands that form saliva and tears are inflamed and stop producing fluid. Your eyes get dry and gritty and your mouth and tongue feel dry. This can lead to scars on the eyes and to difficulty with eating and swallowing. Sometimes glands elsewhere including the gut, lungs and vagina are affected. Sicca syndrome can occur on its own or in combination with rheumatoid arthritis or any of the connective tissue diseases. When it occurs with another disease it is also known as Sjorgrens's syndrome.

## Polymyositis and dermatomyositis

The main problem in these rare diseases is inflammation of muscle, causing pain and weakness. They occasionally complicate any of the other connective tissue diseases, as well as occurring on their own.

## Polyarteritis nodosa

This very rare condition causes patches of inflammation in the walls of blood vessels that can stop the flow of blood. A variety of odd things can occur as a result.

## Common features

There is a good deal of overlap between these diseases. Arthritis can occur in any of them, but this is usually fairly mild and the joints do not become severely damaged or deformed. Another common problem is Raynaud's phenomenon – an abnormality of blood vessels resulting in spasm on exposure to cold. As a result the hands go white and numb for a few moments, before becoming red and painful as the blood flow returns. Raynaud's phenomenon is common, however, and in most cases it occurs on its own and has nothing to do with a connective tissue disease.

## Joint infections

Infection in joints is rare but can occur in three main circumstances:
- Children occasionally get bone infections (osteomyelitis) which then spread to the joints;
- Old people and those with severe illnesses that affect their general resistance to other diseases occasionally get joint infections;
- People with severe rheumatoid arthritis or some other form of advanced joint damage can get an infection on top of the other problems in their joints.

### Types of infection

There are two main types of infection – *acute infections* with bacteria (like those that cause pneumonia and skin boils) and *chronic infections* caused by things like tuberculosis. Bone and joint tuberculosis still occurs occasionally, but most joint infection is of the acute type. Infection should always be considered if someone gets an acute, severe, painful swelling of a joint, especially if they are feverish and ill. But this usually turns out to be something else, like gout!

## Tumours (cancer) in joints

Joint cancer does not occur. Any other part of the body can be affected, however, so it is fascinating that cancer spares the joints. If we could understand why, it might help cancer treatment in general.

### Benign tumours

Just occasionally joints or tendons develop harmless tumour growths. The main type is a condition called 'pigmented villonodular synovitis'. It doesn't spread or cause damage like a cancer and can easily be removed surgically.

# Bone and collagen diseases, and other miscellaneous causes of arthritis

There are many other forms of arthritis, caused by a variety of odd, mostly rare diseases. These can be split into several different types:

### Diseases affecting other parts of the body

Diseases in other parts of the body, particularly if they are near the joints, can cause pain that seems to be due to arthritis. For example, some types of bone disease, including a condition of older people called Paget's disease, cause pains that may seem to come from the joints, even if they don't.

### Bone damage

Bone damage occurring at the end of a long bone next to the joint can cause arthritis directly. One of the most important examples is a condition called 'osteonecrosis', in which a segment of bone dies because its blood flow gets cut off.

### Collagen diseases

Some general diseases of chemicals that help hold our bones, joints and other tissues together can cause arthritis. Collagen is the protein that forms the main fibres of skin, tendons, ligaments and other tough structures in the body. A number of rare abnormalities in its structure occur, resulting in thin, abnormal skin; 'double-jointed', lax joints; and arthritis, among other things.

### A symptom of another disease

Arthritis can occur with, or because of, disease in another part of the body. For example, a glandular abnormality such as thyroid disease can cause pain or swelling of joints. There are many other examples, so 'arthritis' is sometimes the first sign of a quite different type of medical problem.

### Unclassified!

There are still several other odd, rare diseases left, which don't fit any classification, because we don't understand them!

## So what?

Joint pain, or swelling, or both is usually due to an injury or one of the common, mild, periarticular problems mentioned in the next chapter. Sometimes it's caused by one of the major forms of arthritis mentioned in previous chapters. This chapter merely points out that many other conditions can start with or cause joint problems. But don't worry – these problems are rare!

# 10 Periarticular disorders and back pain

As this book is about arthritis, or diseases of joints, it cannot give full coverage to conditions affecting structures outside joints – the periarticular disorders – or to the very common problem of back pain. This chapter aims to provide a brief introduction only to these disorders, pointing out some of the differences between them and arthritis.

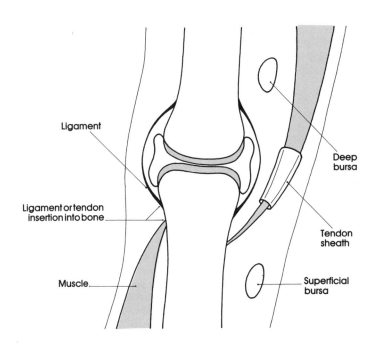

# Periarticular disorders

These are localised, regional disorders, affecting the structures around joints. Most are relatively mild, self-limiting and easy to treat. Other names for these common problems include soft tissue rheumatism, rheumatism, fibrositis and muscular rheumatism. They are quite different from arthritis in several ways. Most importantly they cause no permanant damage and have no lasting effects on joint function.

## Who gets a periarticular problem?

Anyone can! They affect men and women, are rare in childhood and most frequent in middle age. They are very common.

## What are the causes?

The most important cause is overuse or minor injury. Repetitive, unaccustomed activity is a common way of setting off one of these disorders. Occasionally, they are related to one of the arthritic diseases already mentioned, but this is unusual. They often start for no apparent reason.

## What happens?

One of the structures outside the joint is damaged by overuse or injury and this sets up local inflammation at that site. The constant movement that occurs around our joints prevents it settling quickly. The commonest structures to be affected are the bursae, the points at which tendons insert into bone, and the tendons and ligaments themselves.

## Symptoms and signs

The onset is often relatively abrupt. On Monday morning after a 'DIY' weekend, for example, you may wake up with a painful, stiff shoulder. The discomfort is around one joint only, but may seem to cover quite a wide area. It is usually stiff, and certain movements make the pain worse. When the doctor examines you he may find localised, tender spots at the site of damage or he may find some movement or activity that makes it worse.

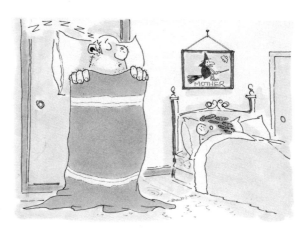

*Odd pains may be due to sleeping in an odd posture.*

This helps sort out exactly which tendon, ligament or bursa is causing the problem.

Rest helps, and these disorders often get better after a few days. Some are more persistent, however, and may take months to settle or need special treatment. They almost always go away eventually, leaving no permanent problems. Recurrences can occur though, especially if you repeat the activity that caused the problem originally. The sportsman prone to tennis elbow or achilles tendonitis, for example, may be at risk throughout his sporting career.

### Complications

There are no complications except for persistent or recurrent episodes in a few unlucky people. Very rarely, there is some permanent damage to a tendon or ligament or minor local damage from recurrent treatment, such as steroid injections causing skin thinning.

### Tests

Tests are unnecessary and unhelpful, but an x-ray is sometimes done to exclude another problem or to rule out a minor fracture after injury.

## Treatment

Rest and time (a few days) are often sufficient, but in persistent cases more help may be needed to speed up recovery (which can take months). There are three main types of treatment:

- Ways of preventing further damage or stress to the affected structure – a splint around the forearm, for example, takes the pressure off the tendons that are inflamed in tennis elbow.
- Local physical treatments – physiotherapists can often help with exercises or ultrasound treatment, which speed up healing.
- Local injections of anaesthetic and steroids (see p. 97) frequently settle these disorders and effect a 'cure'.

## Outcome

Complete recovery with no residual problems occurs in almost all cases.

## Some periarticular disorders

Many of these disorders have amusing names that reflect activities that can cause them. You don't have to be a tennis player, however, to get tennis elbow or a housemaid to get housemaid's knee!

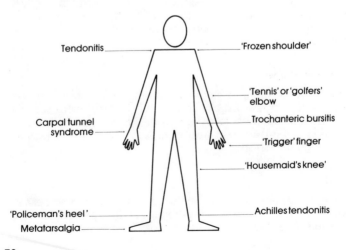

**Frozen shoulder etc.**

Frozen shoulder is a common condition in which one shoulder becomes stiff and painful due to inflammation of the joint capsule. It may take a long time to settle. Tennis and golfer's elbow are caused by inflammation at the site of tendon insertions around the elbow. Trigger finger is a tendonitis of one of the fingers, causing it to get stuck, and then suddenly release, like a trigger. The carpal tunnel syndrome is a little different, however; it is caused by pressure on one of the nerves at the wrist, resulting in pain and tingling in the fingers. Housemaid's knee is a bursitis on the front of the knee. Policeman's heel causes pain under the heel, and is another tendon problem. The Achilles tendon at the back of the heel is also vulnerable, particularly in athletes. Pain under the toes – metatarsalgia – is another common condition. There are many more!

**Fibrositis (muscular rheumatism)**

Fibrositis is a little different. In this condition there is a lot of pain and aching in muscles, especially in the neck and shoulders, which is often worse after activity. Sometimes there is stiffness first thing in the morning, and variable, widespread aching. The pain is not as localised as the conditions mentioned so far. The muscles may be tender to touch, and there may be isolated 'trigger points' of extreme tenderness. Fibrositis is sometimes associated with poor sleep, exhaustion, and sometimes mild depression.

The cause of fibrositis is not known. It seems to be an exaggeration of the everyday muscle aches that we all get from time to time. People who get fibrositis usually go through a bad spell of a few weeks or months, but the condition generally settles, leaving no complications. Treatment is difficult and it is often best to avoid too much in the way of tablets or other specific measures. Plenty of exercise (which won't cause damage even if it hurts) and an active body and mind seem to help it settle more quickly.

## Back pain

Everyone gets back pain – some people get it severely and a few are incapacitated. Backache is an important subject in its own right, with relatively little to do with arthritis.

### Two main types of problem

- Acute back pain – the sudden onset of severe pain in the lower back or neck is common. It usually settles spontaneously after a few days or weeks.
- Chronic back pain – most people get periods of aching or discomfort in parts of their back from time to time, but many suffer this more constantly or more severely than the rest of us. The problem tends to be variable and is related to posture and activity.

### Who gets back pain?

Acute episodes are commonest in young adults, especially those with physically strenuous jobs, whereas chronic pain is more a feature of middle-aged or older adults. It is very common.

### What causes back pain?

Most back pain is mechanical in origin, that is, caused by stresses and strains on the spine. In most cases the pain probably comes from the ligaments, tendons and muscles around the spinal joints and a precise diagnosis is often not possible. But some specific causes are known. These include the prolapse of a disc between the bony vertebrae (slipped disc), osteoarthritis of the small joints (spondylosis), and ankylosing spondylitis. Bone thinning (osteoporosis) is a common problem in older people, especially women, and other bone and joint disorders are occasional causes of back pain.

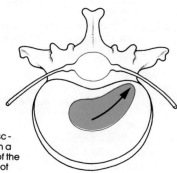

Prolapse of an intervertebral disc - bursting of disc material through a tear in the annulus in the back of the disc and pressing on a nerve root

### What happens?

The problem is commonly a bit like a periarticular disorder. Strain, damage or inflammation of one of the structures in the back causes widespread pain. A secondary problem is muscle spasm, which always seems to follow back pain and makes it worse.

### Symptoms and signs

The pain is often felt around a wide area. There may be one or several areas of tenderness. Spinal movements are usually restricted and painful, partly because of the associated muscle spasm.

### Complications

Complications are rare. Slipped discs occasionally press on nerves, causing damage to muscles and sensation, and bone damage can occur in some of the rarer types of back pain. The consequences of spinal arthritis have been covered in p. 54. The chief complication in most people is simply the frustration, lost time and nuisance value of a 'bad' back.

### Tests

As test results are usually normal they are unhelpful and quite unnecessary in most everyday episodes of acute back pain. A variety of x-ray techniques help the doctor to see the problem in things like slipped discs, and blood tests are occasionally useful to exclude rarer causes.

### Treatment

Rest and time are the most important treatments for most sudden episodes of back pain, but long-standing pain is more difficult to deal with and many different conventional and alternative measures are used to try and help sufferers. In many sudden episodes of pain and for most everyday backaches, mechanical means of treatment are best. These include temporary immobilisation (corsets, collars, and so forth), physiotherapy, and a variety of manipulative techniques. Tablets and injections have only a limited role. In severe, unusual and special situations (such as a slipped disc pressing on a nerve), surgery may be necessary.

**Outcome**

Most acute episodes of back pain settle completely without damage, but a few people get recurrent acute episodes. Those with long-standing back pain usually go through alternating periods of relatively mild and more severe symptoms. The condition often disappears and although long-term damage and disability sometimes occur, these problems are relatively uncommon.

## Painful but not life-threatening!

A fair coverage of back pain needs a book of its own. Back disorders are a major health-care problem today, but most are not associated with any serious disease or arthritis of the spine and do not cause any permanent problems.

# 11 Childhood and Old Age

Although most arthritis begins in young adults or middle-aged people, it can have its onset at the extremes of age both in children and the elderly. The types of arthritis seen at these ages are different from the common disorders of adults. In additon the impact and implications of arthritis are quite different in childhood and old age.

## Arthritis in children

Lots of children get aches and pains in their muscles and joints but true arthritis is rare.

### Childhood joint pains

Limb pains ('growing pains') occur in about 5% of children. Their cause is unknown and they have no long-term importance. Viral infections are a common cause of short-lasting muscle and joint pains. Injury is the other common cause, and some children, especially those who are particularly loose-limbed (hypermobile, or 'double-jointed'), get frequent aches and pains after exercise or minor injuries. Short-lasting hip problems (the 'irritable hip syndrome') and other regional disorders of a more specific nature sometimes occur. Attention-seeking behaviour, undisclosed injuries (battering), and rare childhood diseases occasionally present as 'arthritis'.

### Childhood arthritis

There is a small number of specific arthritic diseases of children. Rheumatic fever used to be the commonest cause, but fortunately this condition is now quite rare in most developed countries. Most childhood arthritis seen today comes under the umbrella diagnosis of *'juvenile chronic arthritis'*. Other arthritic diseases occuring in children are very rare.

Juvenile chronic arthritis is the term used to describe pain and swelling of one or more joints which persists for longer than three months in people under 16 years old. It can take several forms. The commonest type affects only a few joints and grumbles on for several years. Another type is more like rheumatoid arthritis and can cause severe, widespread joint damage. The third main form used to be called Still's disease (after Sir George Fredrick Still who described it), and causes fevers, rashes and other general problems as well as arthritis. Most cases burn out as the children grow older, but they can cause a lot of pain, suffering and deformity.

### Children with arthritis

Arthritis is no fun at any age. But children face special problems. Any condition which makes it hard for children to get about or join in games causes great psychological problems as well as physical ones. Arthritis occurring during growth can affect development, sometimes resulting in deformity, short stature, or uneven growth of limbs or digits. Children with arthritis need special care and attention, both for the disease itself and to minimise the lasting physical and psychological scars.

## Arthritis in the elderly

Arthritis and rheumatism are the commonest cause of disability in the elderly. There are several reasons for this. Most rheumatic diseases don't kill, so that the cumulative effect of more and more people getting arthritis at different times of life means that it is commonest in old people. Secondly, it gets much more difficult to cope with arthritis as you get older, particularly if you have other problems with balance, sight, or hearing, for example. Ageing bones and muscles, as well as social and psychological problems, often add to the burden.

### Joint pains in the elderly

Aches and pains of some sort are almost universal in older people, and accepted by most as a part of ageing. Mostly they are not due to arthritis. The periarticular and back problems described in chapter 1 and 'fibrositis' ('muscular rheumatism') are very common in the elderly. Minor injuries, postural problems, awkward movements, and muscular weakness and stiffness can all cause pain. Some other diseases of older people, like Parkinson's disease, can also cause muscle and joint pains simulating 'arthritis'.

Ageing causes the muscles to weaken, the bones to get

thinner, and the joints to get stiffer. Older people move about more slowly and can do less physical activity than the young. But despite this, most function well and don't have severe arthritis.

### Arthritis of the elderly

Although many of the major rheumatic diseases can begin in older people, the 'sero-negative spondarthritis group' rarely do so. Osteoarthritis and some crystal-related arthritis are however, particularly common. There are also a few special forms of arthritis that are only seen in the elderly – for example, an uncommon form of severe joint destruction, occuring at the shoulders, knees and some other joints.

### Polymyalgia rheumatica

This is another important condition of the elderly, characterised by pain and stiffness around the shoulders and hips. There is usually severe stiffness in the morning, and sufferers often have the greatest of difficulty in getting out of bed. They usually feel rotten and depressed, and may have mild fevers and other limb pains as well. It is sometimes associated with inflammation in blood vessels that can be dangerous, occasionally causing strokes or blindness. Fortunately polymyalgia rheumatica responds quickly and well to small doses of steroid tablets. This treatment also prevents the blood vessel problems.

### The elderly arthritic

Just as children have special needs, so do the elderly. As we age we loose some of the ability to adapt to changes, including things like developing arthritis. Many old people become isolated and depressed, particularly if they are physically handicapped. Treatment is more difficult than in younger people; drugs need special care and immobility is especially dangerous. Constant pain and stiffness may be a dreadful burden on top of all the other disadvantages of age. Elderly people with arthritis should command our special respect and care.

# 12 Can arthritis be treated?

Arthritis often gets better... but it requires help. Help from the sufferer, who needs to have the right attitude and approach to the problem, is particularly important. Help from doctors and therapists is also valuable.

## Remission

Many forms of arthritis get better on their own, given time. This is natural *remission* and it has nothing to do with treatment. If a condition goes into remission when the sufferer is trying a special treatment, false claims about some new therapy can arise.

### Cure

Some diseases, including a few forms of arthritis, can be cured. This means that there is a specific treatment for the condition, that either gets rid of the cause or gets rid of the effects so successfully that the disease process is stopped. Many infections, including those in joints, can be cured by modern antibiotics. However, the result obviously depends on whether or not irreparable damage was done by the disease (or its treatment) beforehand.

### Treatment

Most arthritic diseases can be treated but not cured. Treatment can control a disease so well that it is no longer a problem. High blood pressure, for example, can be kept normal with tablets, preventing the problems it might otherwise cause. This is a very effective therapy. The degree of success of treatment for rheumatic diseases varies: it is often, but not always, good. Most arthritis isn't as simple as high blood pressure, although the treatment of gout is excellent. But even if effective disease control is not possible, treatment can help relieve symptoms and suffering. A great deal can be achieved by simple measures and common sense as outlined in some of the chapters that follow.

There is always some treatment available to an arthritis sufferer. If he or she is lucky there may be a cure, or at least a highly effective way of controlling the disease. If not, treatment can help relieve suffering. There is also the hope that comes with the knowledge that natural remission can occur at any time.

## An age-old problem

There is nothing new about arthritis or its treatment. Old skeletons show that our ancestors often had arthritis and old medical and non-medical writings testify to the suffering it caused, and the attempts to treat it.

### Warmth, embrocations . . . and needles

It has been known for centuries that warmth, local rubs and applications, and bathing can ease rheumatic pains and arthritis. Numerous different things have been rubbed into or wrapped around painful joints over the centuries. Spas were famous for the relief they provided and 'hydrotherapy' remains important today. The idea that diet is important is also old, and many types of diet have been recommended. There have probably been as many claims for a dietary 'cure' as there are types of rheumatism and arthritis! All sorts of other ways of soothing painful joints and helping arthritis have been invented from Chinese acupuncture to modern pain clinics; from stretching on the 'rack' to osteopathy and chiropracter. These and many others all have a place.

### Improvements

Treatment is getting better. New drugs and operations are safer and more effective than before and there is also greater recognition of what can be achieved through self-help and caring. The best of the old is being combined with modern therapy to improve the lot of the arthritis sufferer and provide a more rounded, holistic approach to treatment. But there is still a long way to go, both in awareness and understanding.

## Aims and objectives

There are three main objectives in treating arthritis:
- Relief of pain and suffering;
- Maintenance of maximum function and independence;
- Treatment of the disease process.

Their order and importance varies in different stages of a disease, in different people and in the different types of arthritis. In addition, a particular type of treatment may meet more than one of the three main aims – relief of pain, for example, may lead to improved function.

## Types of treatment available

All sorts of different types of treatment are available. It is impossible to do them all justice in this book, but some of the more important and widely used approaches are covered in the next chapters.

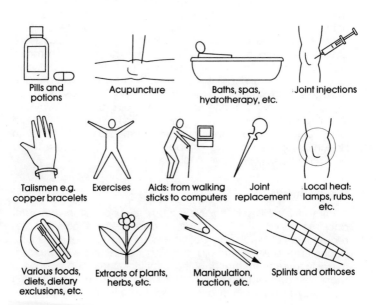

Pills and potions

Acupuncture

Baths, spas, hydrotherapy, etc.

Joint injections

Talismen e.g. copper bracelets

Exercises

Aids: from walking sticks to computers

Joint replacement

Local heat: lamps, rubs, etc.

Various foods, diets, dietary exclusions, etc.

Extracts of plants, herbs, etc.

Manipulation, traction, etc.

Splints and orthoses

### Right mental approach

Understanding the problem makes it easier to cope with. Sufferers and their relatives need to know about their arthritis and have some idea of how best to help themselves.

The right mental approach is important. You should be philosophical about arthritis and respect it, but not give in to it or let it get on top of you. You also need to find the right balance of rest and exercise.

### Help from therapists

The professional help and advice available from the physiotherapists and occupational therapists is often invaluable in helping people to help themselves, protect their joints and live easier lives.

Specific exercises and local applications are also the province of the therapists. Physiotherapists help maintain and improve strength, movement and function. Pain relief is sometimes achieved through *manipulation*, which is also done by osteopaths and chiropracters, and can be particularly helpful for back pain.

### Aids and appliances

Various aids and appliances can improve function and increase the independence of people with some physical disability. The occupational therapist has a range of ingenious skills, strategies and devices, often very simple, which can help enormously. They range from shoes and splints to walking aids, bath and toilet aids, or complex computerised systems for the severely handicapped.

### Drugs and surgery

These are providing more and more advantages as they improve. A whole range of different injections, pills, operations and procedures is now available.

### Alternative approaches

A variety of experimental and unproved treatments are in use, some by alternative practitioners, some in scientific studies in hospitals or universities. Alternative medicine is widely used for arthritis; but it's no longer so 'alternative'. There is increasing dialogue between traditional and unusual forms of medicine, and increasing incorporation of the 'best of everything' into the total caring of arthritis. Doctors are researching into diets as well as drugs, and into the effects of things like acupuncture as well as surgery.

## Something for everyone

Some things help one patient, other things work for another. There are very few sufferers who can't get a good deal of help from some or several of the available measures to treat arthritis.

# 13 Drugs, injections and therapists

About drugs

## About drugs

Drug treatment has an important place in helping arthritis, but like most things it needs to be tailored to your needs and integrated with all other aspects of treatment.

Most people with serious arthritis take drugs regularly, and most are much better for it. Drugs often make the difference between being able to get out and about or being stuck at home. A few people get side effects, however, and a small minority either have serious side effects or don't seem to get any benefit from drugs. Unfortunately, these problems often get more publicity than the benefits and, as a result, many of us have mixed feelings – we realise that drugs can be very beneficial, but we are a bit scared of taking them.

### What is a drug?

'Drugs' are everywhere – in things like tea, coffee, beer, plants and trees. They are chemicals that can have a specific effect on some aspect of the body's function, and many of those used today come from natural sources such as plants. The difference between the tablet you take and the tea you drink is that the tablet contains a concentrated, purified form of a specific chemical, whereas tea contains small amounts of several chemicals.

### Individual variations

Drugs don't always work in exactly the same way in everyone. One person might find aspirin marvellous for their headaches while another may find that it does nothing except give them tummy ache. The problem is no drug is entirely predictable.

### Risks against benefits

No drug is perfectly safe for everyone. But no day is perfectly safe either – we all take risks all the time. Just like everything else, taking a drug is to take a calculated risk, but in most cases the risk is tiny, certainly much less than the risk of surgery and probably less than that of going on long car journeys. The more powerful and effective a drug, however, the greater the risks. So some of the drugs used for severe, advanced arthritis carry a higher risk and may need careful monitoring. Doctors, drug companies and licensing authorities are all very concerned with the risk: benefit ratio of drugs.

---

**The chances that it will do good have to outweigh massively the risk of side effects before a drug is licensed.**

---

### Drugs for arthritis

Four main types of drug are used in the treatment of arthritis:
- Pain killers;
- Anti-inflammatory agents:
- Steroids;
- Drugs that control or modify specific arthritic diseases.

## Pain killers

Pain killers don't kill pain – they reduce it, dull it, 'take the edge off', but do nothing to treat the underlying cause of the pain. Pain killers work by blocking the transmission of pain signals to the brain. Some work more at the site of the problem, others work more on the brain itself. Most work for only a few hours and then get washed out of the system by the kidneys.

### Side effects

Pain killers may have side effects. They can reduce the transmission of other signals around the nervous system, as well as pain pathways and as a result, some cause drowsiness. Other things, such as alcohol, that can depress nervous function may accentuate the effects of these drugs. Pain killers can also affect the way your bowel works causing constipation. Strong pain killers like morphine are addictive.

## Examples

Simple, mild pain killers like aspirin, paracetamol and codeine are available at chemists without prescription. A few slightly stronger ones such as dextropropoxyphene are often prescribed for arthritis, but strong, addictive drugs like pethidine and morphine are hardly ever used. Mixtures of small doses of two or three pain killers sometimes seem to work better than one on its own and many of the prescribed and 'over the counter' preparations are mixtures.

## Their use in arthritis

Most pain killers work for only a few hours. It is often wisest to limit their use to times when pain is particularly bad or before doing something that has to be done but you know will cause pain. Some unfortunate people need regular pain killers in addition to other treatments to make life bearable.

## Anti-inflammatory agents

These drugs reduce inflammation anywhere in the body. They don't alter the cause or the disease, but by reducing inflammation they reduce pain, swelling and stiffness. If your arthritis is an inflammatory sort, like rheumatoid arthritis, they may be much more effective in pain control than pain killers.

Most anti-inflammatory drugs seem to work by interfering with one specific chemical which is central to inflammation – an enzyme called cyclo-oxygenase. This action reduces the effects of inflammation, including pain.

## Side effects

Anti-inflammatory drugs may cause indigestion and occasionally ulcers. Other rare side effects are fluid retention, rashes and drowsiness. Fortunately, side effects are uncommon and usually mild, but they are more of a problem in elderly people, in whom these drugs have to be used particularly cautiously.

## Examples

There are several anti-inflammatory drugs. High-dose aspirin has an anti-inflammatory effect, but most modern drugs used for arthritis are safer and less likely to cause side effects than large doses of aspirin. The many different drugs all have much the same effect, although some work better than others for any individual. Most need to be taken only once or twice a day, but several days of regular use are needed to achieve the best results. Examples include Brufen (ibuprofen), Naprosyn (naproxen), Voltarol (diclofenac), Feldene (piroxicam), Indocid (indomethacin). (All drugs have three different names: a chemical name that is usually long and cumbersome, a registered name of the compound, and a licensed name used by a company who makes and markets it. In this instance I have used the licensed company name first with the registered 'proper' name in brackets.)

## Their use in arthritis

If you have an inflammatory form of arthritis try one of these drugs, and if it doesn't suit you try another. Each one should be tried for a couple of weeks to see if it works. They often produce extensive reduction of pain and stiffness and a dose last thing at night may reduce difficulties in the morning. Your doctor will advise you of the best dose and drug for your needs. These drugs are less useful in rheumatism and osteo-arthritis, but are sometimes worth trying. If you are not sure of their value after a time using them, try without for a week and keep a note of the difference. Always be sure that the drug is doing something positive before going on with regular use.

## Steroids

Steroids, including cortisone, are a group of natural body hormones that have numerous effects on the body's metabolism. They help keep our bones and skin healthy and affect practically all of our organs. Their main value in arthritis is their ability to reduce inflammation and damp down the body's immune defence reactions.

Steroids affect all sorts of metabolic reactions in the body and by giving extra (in tablets or by injection) the balance is changed a bit. One of the things that extra steroids do is help block excess inflammation, by a mechanism similar to that of the drugs mentioned in the previous section.

### Side effects

Because steroids control body metabolism, extra doses given for long periods can have all sorts of adverse side effects. They can cause thinning of bones and skin, excess body fat, increased blood pressure, fluid retention, cataracts, and other things. All these problems depend on the dose used, however, and the length of time steroids are taken for. Small doses can provide benefits without side effects. Steroids need to be carefully controlled. The body gets used to the extra doses and if you have been on steroids for a while it is dangerous to reduce the dose too quickly.

### Their use in arthritis

There are a few disorders in which steroids are essential to prevent serious problems and even loss of life. These include polymyalgia rheumatica and arteritis, and severe flare-ups of systemic lupus erythematosis and other connective tissue diseases. In other severe inflammatory forms of arthritis they can be valuable either for short periods to get things under control, or in low doses. Steroids are also useful for injection into joints.

## Disease-modifying agents

These drugs have some fundamental effect on the cause of the arthritis, slowing down or preventing damage. They often take a long time to work, so it may be weeks or months before you feel better. When they work well, however, the results can be dramatic, with a considerable improvement in all aspects of the arthritis.

Drugs for gout work by keeping uric acid levels low and some of the others seem to suppress immune reactions in the body. For most disease-modifying agents used for rheumatoid and other forms of arthritis, however, we don't yet know how they work.

### Side effects

Gout drugs are very safe but most of the others can cause problems. Although damage to the blood or the kidney as well as rashes and indigestion can occur, these and other side effects nearly always go away completely when the drugs are stopped. Many of these drugs have to be monitored carefully, with regular blood or urine tests or both to check that all is well.

### Examples

Gout drugs are dealt with on p. 66. The others fall into two main categories: the so-called 'immunosuppressive agents' which include azathioprine, methotrexate and cyclophosphamide and a miscellaneous group which affect rheumatoid and other forms of arthritis and include gold, d-penicillamine, hydroxy-chloroquine and sulphasalazine.

### Their use in arthritis

These drugs should be used carefully in arthritis, with a doctor controlling and supervising treatment at regular intervals. There are no simple rules about when and which drug; you must rely on your doctor or specialist to discuss this with you and give advice.

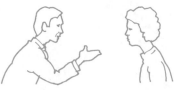

## Problems and responsibility

In order to get the benefits, whilst minimising the risks, everyone involved must take responsibility for drug usage. Drug companies need to be as careful as they can about testing the agents and providing doctors and pharmacists with the right information. They, in turn must be cautious in prescribing and monitoring drug usage. Both activities are supervised by the regulatory bodies such as Britain's 'Committee for the Safety of Medicines'. But it doesn't stop there: sensible drug usage is also the responsibility of the person taking the drug.

## Injections

Injections allow delivery of effective medicines to the place they are needed, without the whole body being affected. Local injections into or around joints are widely used in the treatment of arthritis and rheumatism.

### Medicines given by injection

The main drugs used in this way are steroids. Special forms have been produced that stay at the site of injection. Very little gets absorbed into the circulation, so relatively large doses can be given, resulting in an effective but temporary relief of local inflammation with few side effects.

Other drugs, designed to produce more lasting results, are occasionally used, ranging from acids, which literally burn out the inflamed tissue, to radioactive compounds that deliver a small, localised dose of irradiation to kill the arthritic inflammation.

Local anaesthetics are often used in combination with these other drugs for pain relief.

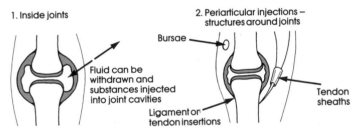

**Injections for arthritis and tendon injuries.**

### Injections for periarticular rheumatism

Many forms of periarticular rheumatism are caused by inflammation at the site of a tendon, ligament or bursa. Local injections to the inflamed area can be very effective. Although the drug effect lasts for only a few weeks, this can be sufficient to 'cure' the condition provided that the person doesn't repeat the sort of misuse that started it. Injections are a good way of treating many common, minor forms of rheumatism like tennis elbow and some shoulder problems.

### Injections into joints for arthritis

Most joints can be injected relatively easily and painlessly by experts. Very tense, swollen joints can be relieved by removal of excess joint fluid (aspiration) to reduce the painful pressure in the joint. At the same time steroids, or longer-acting anti-inflammatory agents, can be injected into the joint to stop the fluid coming straight back again. This is a useful way of treating an inflammatory flare-up of a joint affected by arthritis. The effect lasts for a variable time, depending on a number of things including the activity of the disease. Sometimes people get good relief for months or even years, on other occasions it lasts for only a few days or weeks.

### Used in combination

Injections of this sort are often used in combination with other treatments. For example, temporary relief of pain and pressure in a joint may help the physiotherapist work on the muscles and movements to get a limb going again. They are also used to give long-suffering patients and joints a 'holiday' from the pain. But they can't be used too often. The risks of one injection are very small, but too many too often can occasionally contribute to more joint damage or predispose the joint to infection. Injection treatment is also limited because it is impossible to use it on more than one or two joints at a time; it is no solution for a patient with generalised arthritis.

Joint injections then are a useful addition to other treatment, but, like everything else, need caution and sensible use.

## The therapists

Spas, splints, massage and many other forms of 'physical therapy' have been in use for centuries. Nor is there anything new in helping people to lead independent lives in spite of physical handicap. These approaches to treatment are now largely the province of the 'therapists' – specially trained professionals skilled in the assessment and treatment of physical disability.

## Physiotherapists

Physiotherapists are trained in the assessment and physical treatment of disorders of the musculoskeletal system. They use several different methods to reduce pain, improve strength and movement, and increase function. These include special exercises, mobilising and manipulating joints, hydrotherapy (exercises in warm water) and the application of a number of soothing treatments such as heat or ice packs. Other equipment used by physiotherapists, such as ultrasound machines, may help muscles, ligaments and tendons to heal after injury.

## Occupational therapists

Occupational therapists are more concerned with the way people manage at home and in the community. Their special training helps them to perform a detailed functional assessment of everyday tasks such as washing, dressing, cooking and cleaning. They can also examine people's ability to cope with their work. They may visit patients at home and provide an important link between hospital-based services and the community. The occupational therapist can advise about ways of reducing stress, both physical and mental; provide aids to improve independence; counsel people about coping with physical disability; and liaise with social workers and others at the community level.

## Orthotists and chiropodists

Orthotists make splints and appliances to help in the job of reducing pain and improving function. Splints rest inflamed joints and support unstable ones. A variety of walking aids are available and special shoes for painful deformed feet can be a great help. The *chiropodist* also takes a special interest in feet, and can help treat painful corns, bunions and many other foot problems.

## A team

The treatment of physical disability caused by joint disorders requires a coordinated team approach, making full use of the varied and considerable skills of the therapists and others. Doctors often find themselves helping in the coordination of therapists, nurses, social workers and others. In many instances finding the right member of the team to do the job is more important than pills, potions or alternative medicines.

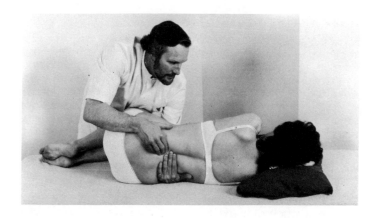

**What do the therapists do?**

The job of any of the people in the team can be broken down into a few simple headings:
- Assessment;
- Finding physical means of reducing pain;
- Improving function;
- Communicating with the patient, his or her family, and other members of the treatment team.

*Assessment* This is a vital part of the work of all therapists. A full assessment of the problems of someone with arthritis may take more than an hour; but if it leads to a clearer understanding of the complex interaction of physical, psychological and social problems it can be immensely valuable in itself. A good assessment of the problem often makes the answers obvious.

*Relieving symptoms* Pain can be eased by the local application of heat as well as exercises and a variety of other physical methods. Help in muscle relaxation and education in the use of muscles and joints can also do much to relieve pain. Acutely inflamed joints may need support and rest in splints. The therapist may also be able to teach a regime of limbering-up exercises to relieve stiffness. If symptoms are caused by some mechanical abnormality, such as leg shortening or some particular way of using the back or limbs, the therapist may be able to help diagnose and solve the problem.

*Improving function* Helping disabled people to improve function and live more independent lives often requires all the skills and ingenuity of the therapists. It involves the use of many different methods ranging from education and exercises to complex aids and appliances. The physiotherapist can help muscles to maintain or regain strength, improve the range of motion of joints, and re-educate the body to function better. The occupational therapist can help apply this improvement in physical ability to the person's situation at work and at home. The help of other health-care professionals such as nurses, health visitors and social workers may also be needed in difficult cases.

*Vital work* It is impossible to do justice to the vital work of the therapists here. They are carrying on a tradition of physical and social support for disabled and arthritic people that goes back centuries. Therapists are now extending that work, and inter-relating it with the current scientific advances in medicine and the increased social awareness of disability and the needs of the handicapped.

*Aids such as wide handled cutlery make life a lot easier.*

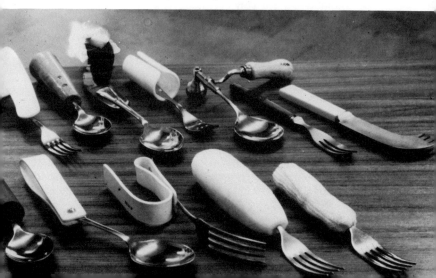

# 14 Surgery

Arthritis surgery has advanced tremendously in recent years and techniques such as the replacement of destroyed joints have eased the lives of many people. Although a wide range of different operations is used in the treatment of joint disease; most people with arthritis will never need any of them, as surgery is indicated in only a few specific instances in the more serious forms of arthritis.

## Which diseases might need surgery?

Severe rheumatoid arthritis and osteoarthritis are most likely to need surgery. Occasionally people with ankylosing spondylitis need operations on their spine or hips, and a few people with psoriatic arthritis and some of the other less common forms of joint disease may also have surgery. Sufferers from gout, those with milder forms of rheumatoid and osteoarthritis, people with the connective tissue diseases, and most of those with back and periarticular problems will never need an operation. Overall the proportion of arthritis patients having surgery for their joint disease is very small.

## What types of operation are there?

The operations, like the diseases, can be divided into periarticular (outside the joint itself) and articular (on the joint proper). Periarticular surgery is usually relatively minor and includes the repair of damaged tendons and ligaments and the removal of large cysts and nodules. Articular surgery can be divided further into four main types:

## Synovectomy

The lining of the joint (the synovium) is sometimes removed surgically if it is very bulky and inflamed. Synovectomy is not common, but can be useful if the bulky synovium is causing mechanical problems or threatening to damage tendons and ligaments.

## Arthrodesis

A joint can be fixed permanently, either by bone grafting, or by nailing or wiring the two halves together. This is called an arthrodesis and is sometimes used to help a joint which is already restricted in movement but very painful. An arthrodesed joint can't move, but it is not painful.

## Osteotomy

Osteotomy is an operation where the bone next to a painful joint is cut then refixed in a slightly different position. This operation is used to correct deformity and relieve pain in osteoarthritis, mostly of the knee or foot. It can also stimulate the joint to heal.

## Joint replacement

Joint replacements are now commonplace. Before artificial joints (prostheses) were available, the only option other than arthrodesis was to cut part of the joint out. This is called an excision arthroplasty and is rarely necessary today. Modern metal alloy and high density plastics have allowed artificial joints to be developed for many different sites. Hips were first and remain the most reliable but knee replacements are rapidly catching up. Prostheses are also available for the small joints of the hand, the shoulder, elbow and ankle.

Artificial joints are not perfect. They don't function as well as a natural joint, and may not last longer than 15 years or so. Furthermore, in about one case in 20, the operation doesn't work perfectly and some complication spoils the success. So the decision to put in a new joint is not taken lightly and the risks have to be carefully weighed up against the likely benefit in every case. Nevertheless, there are many people today who are delighted with their new joints and the demand is increasing. A good joint replacement provides an adequate range of movement for most everyday activity without pain.

# Which joints can be operated on?

Nearly everything *can* be operated on, but only a few procedures are commonly used. Only some of the most popular operations can be mentioned below.

### The hip

Hip replacement is so successful that it has overtaken all other procedures. Severe pain and disability that do not respond to other treatment may be an indication for a new joint.

### The knee

Surgeons often explore the knee through a small telescope called an arthroscope. Minor operations can be performed through this instrument, which also allows the inside of the knee to be visualised so that the diagnosis can be made. A biopsy of the lining is sometimes useful when trying to find out the cause of knee problems. In advanced osteoarthritis an osteotomy can be very helpful, but the severely damaged rheumatoid knee may need replacement. There is sometimes a need for synovectomy or the removal of cysts in the knee.

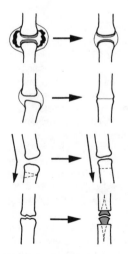

1. Synovectomy
A thick inflamed joint lining is removed

2. Arthrodesis (fusion)
An unstable joint is fused – the bones are fixed together

3. Osteotomy
An angulated deformity of a joint is corrected by taking a 'wedge' of bone out. This operation also relieves pain

4. Arthroplasty (replacement)
A damaged joint is replaced by an artificial one made of metal or plastic

**Types of operations.**

### The hand

Hand surgery is particularly delicate and specialised. Many different operations are available, including tendon release and repair, decompression of trapped nerves, fixation for the painful wrist, and small joint replacements. Hand surgeons often work closely with occupational therapists and other doctors so that hand function can be carefully assessed in the light of all other problems before embarking on any procedure. Maintaining hand function is regarded as the main concern.

### The spine

Back surgery is also a large, specialist area. Some operations are done by neurosurgeons as well as orthopaedic surgeons. Removal of 'slipped discs' is the best known operation, but fixation (arthrodesis) and other types of procedure are also available.

### The foot

One of the most useful operations for people with bad rheumatoid arthritis involves cutting out damaged joints at the base of the toes to allow them to walk without pain again. 'Bunion' operations are also popular and a variety of other operations on the ankle area can be useful.

### Shoulders and elbows

Joint replacement has been slower to develop for these two joints, but improvements are coming along and surgical help is available for those with terrible pain and damage at these sites.

## When is surgery recommended?

Surgery for arthritis must be integrated with all other aspects of patient management. Many hospitals run 'combined clinics' attended by a medical specialist (a rheumatologist), an orthopaedic surgeon and therapists. The problems are discussed openly so that any decision to recommend surgery is one that everyone feels happy with, including the patient! These decisions are not easy. If several joints are affected it can be hard to predict the benefit of operating on one of them. Other things that must be taken into account include any medical treatment and the activity of the disease. One of the most difficult tasks is to recommend the right operation at the right time.

> **Surgery is not a last resort. It is an important means of treating bad arthritis. The right operation, done at the right time in conjunction with other aspects of treatment, can be tremendously helpful.**

# 15 Alternative complementary medicine

Over recent years conventional medicine has become more 'holistic' than ever before. In other words doctors are fully aware of the need for total patient care, which takes all aspects of a person's needs into account. In addition, many of the approaches used by alternative practitioners have become incorporated into everyday medical practice. A preferred term for many of the treatments discussed below is 'complementary medicine'.

## Differences between traditional and alternative medicine

The main differences between traditional and alternative medicine today are:

### Legal control

There is no legal control over alternative medicine. A doctor's training and practice are under strict professional surveillance and although this is true of some forms of alternative medicine, it is not true for all. Unfortunately, there are practitioners who have little or no training and whose work is questionable, and it is often difficult for patients to know who does and does not have appropriate qualifications.

### Safety and effectiveness

There is no requirement to test either the effectiveness or safety of alternative medicine, whereas any form of treatment offered within the conventional health system has been rigorously tested for both its safety and its ability to work better than a dummy treatment (placebo). Many forms of alternative medicine are both safe and helpful, but these differences make it a difficult area for both patients and doctors.

## Special problems in arthritis

Alternative medicine for things like arthritis presents other, special problems. Throughout this book the variability and unpredictability of most forms of arthritis have been stressed and it is also true that our present conventional treatments are far from perfect. As a result of this many people use untried, alternative therapy, with a mixture of success, apparent success, failure or side effects. Sorting out what is due to a placebo effect, what improvements are a result of the condition going into natural remission and what is due to a medicine is very difficult. Also, as a result of one person's experience, exaggerated claims are often made, and because people are desperate for help, they will often try anything. Sadly they are often bitterly disappointed.

It is impossible to do justice to all forms of alternative medicine in this book. I have split them into those allied to or used in traditional medicine, and those that remain more removed from a conventional doctor's approach.

## Alternative therapies related to conventional medicine

### Spas, mud and water

Spa treatment has been used in arthritis for many centuries. Local warmth, be it via water, mud packs or anything else, relieves pain and stiffness and helps get muscles and joints moving. Immersion in water has beneficial physiological effects and because gravity is lessened, it also helps disabled people get moving. There is however, no evidence that spa or mineral waters are any better than a physiotherapist's hydrotherapy pool.

### Acupuncture and pain control

Chinese acupuncture can relieve pain. Unfortunately the effect usually doesn't last for very long and there is no reason to believe that acupuncture has any effect on arthritic diseases. Nevertheless, this and other physical forms of pain control are now being used with conventional medicine.

## Osteopathy and manipulation

Physical manipulation of bones and joints is another form of treatment with a long history. It is now used by physiotherapists, doctors, osteopaths, chiropracters and others. It can be very valuable, particularly in the treatment of some forms of back pain, but some caution is needed. Inflammatory diseases can be made worse by manipulation, and if arthritis has already caused damage, this therapy can be dangerous. It is important to be sure of the diagnosis first.

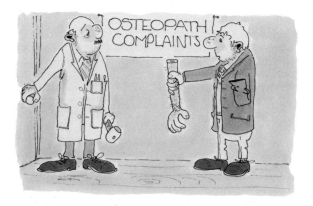

*Manipulation may sometimes be dangerous.*

## Homoeopathy

Homoeopathy uses very small quantities of certain chemicals to treat individual patients and problems. Most practitioners also have a conventional medical degree and often use both forms of treatment. Attempts have been made to test homoeopathy in arthritis formally, but the results have not been very encouraging.

## Rubs, sprays, lotions etc.

Rubbing things into joints is another ancient, popular approach to treating arthritis. Large numbers of 'rubrifacients' are available from chemists and elsewhere. Most of them provide *temporary* pain relief, but don't seem to do anything else.

### Dietary treatment

A huge number of different diets are recommended for arthritis. Book shops and magazines are full of special diets – all of them different. This subject probably causes arthritis sufferers as much anxiety (and often money) as any other.

Most people with a major form of arthritis don't seem to be any different whatever diet they try. (If there were a simple answer we would all know it and there would only be one book on the shelves!) A few arthritics and some people with recurrent aches and pain do, however, seem to be sensitive to some foods. There is no clear pattern or way of predicting this and allergy tests don't help so it is difficult to give individual advice.

However, two different aspects of dietary treatment of arthritis are currently being investigated by doctors and dieticians. A few people with inflammatory arthritis seem to improve with removal of certain foods from the diet and a variety of exclusion diets are being researched. More promising, is the use of different fats in the diet, such as fish oil and Evening Primrose. These substances alter the type of chemical produced by the body during an inflammatory response. They may help relieve symptoms if used in conjunction with other means of reducing inflammation. A lot of research is being done to sort out how useful this sort of dietary treatment might be, and how best to use it.

## Treatments not used with conventional medicine

### Herbal medicine

Many very important drugs have come from plants and herbs. The use of herbs and other vegetable extracts remains as popular today as ever, but this form of treatment is not part of conventional medicine because there is no reason to think that it does much good (or harm).

### Allergy treatments

Most forms of arthritis have nothing to do with allergy. Many other disorders, such as hay fever and nettle rash, are allergies, and allergy clinics and treatments are a part of conventional medicine. But there are also numbers of alternative practitioners doing dubious allergy tests and recommending strange forms of treatment for arthritis, for which there is no apparent basis.

### Reflexology and allied disciplines

It seems highly unlikely that these approaches, based on a claimed representation of different parts of the body on the soles of the feet, have anything to offer people with arthritis.

### Talismen

Lots of us believe in a lucky charm or carry something around 'for luck'. Many such objects have been claimed to help arthritis over the years. Copper bangles are a current favourite, but again there is no evidence to suggest they do much.

### Green lipped mussels and allied treatments

A few years ago capsules containing an extract from the green lipped mussel (which comes from New Zealand) were first marketed as a 'cure' for arthritis. This is one of many such false claims made from time to time for some unlikely treatment. It is impossible to list all the different remedies that are being sold for arthritis; suffice it to say that doctors are already using any that have proven benefit and no serious side effects.

## Conclusions

Many forms of alternative medicine are safe and effective. Most of these are well known to conventional doctors and some are now used in hospital medicine. Others are either ineffective, dangerous, expensive, or all three. So do combine any form of alternative medicine with the conventional approach and ask your doctor for advice.

# 16 Self-help and living with disability

This chapter concerns the ways in which people with arthritis can help themselves, as well as strategies for coping with disability and handicap. Inevitably the advice given will be of more relevance to some than others and can be only of a very general nature. Your doctor or therapist may be able to help more with specific advice for you. It is obviously important to find out how best to help yourself.

Arthritis sufferers are bombarded with suggestions and advice from well-meaning friends and relatives, as well as by media stories, many of which are distorted. Much of this advice is inappropriate, sometimes it is incorrect. Furthermore, different things suit different people and different diseases. It is a wonderful tribute to most of you with severe arthritis, that you find your way through the jungle of conflicting advice and learn how to cope.

## Becoming an 'arthritic'

Getting arthritis has been likened to a bereavement. The loss of a part of your physical prowess, a part of yourself, is like losing a loved one. At first there is the shock; then the anger and resentment – 'why me?'; next comes the depression and frustration; finally you find your way to accepting the situation for what it is.

### Coming to terms with arthritis

The sooner you can accept it the better. Many people with arthritis are stuck with it. It may not be a disaster and treatment may be controlling it, but they know it will always be part of them. It is important that you come to terms with this. Talking about it, learning about it, even crying about it, may help. This does not mean giving in to arthritis, far from it. What it means is that you accept the presence of the disease, enjoy life within your limitations, and look forward to what can be done rather than looking back at what might have been.

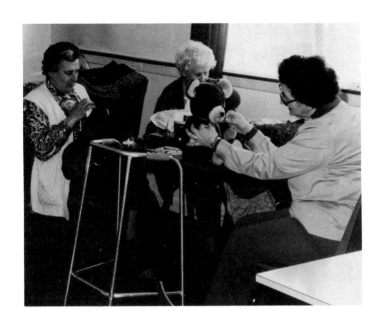

*Enjoy life within your limitations.*

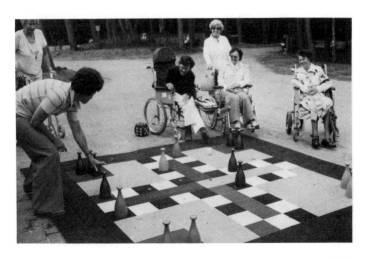

**It's no picnic . . . but**

Having arthritis is 'no picnic'. You may have pain, you may feel awful at times, you may think you look awful, and you may not be able to do things as you would like. But you musn't let it become a disaster. No-one is interested in your becoming a martyr to arthritis. For a full and fulfilling future you need to relax into it, find ways round the problems, keep up with your family and friends, and keep smiling. Talk about arthritis, share it with others but never let it take over.

## Relaxation

Tension is destructive. It knots up your muscles and makes them hurt, it grinds joints together, and it makes you more tired and irritable. If stress, tension and frustration are stopping you from sleeping properly the problem just gets worse and worse. Rule number one in fighting arthritis is *fight against tension*. Learn to relax. For many of you that means learning a new and important skill. Once you get the hang of it, it's easy, for ever remembered and very valuable. This may mean 20 minutes or so of your time once or twice a day but the benefits can be tremendous.

**How to relax**

- Find a quiet place where you can lie down comfortably and forget about everything around you as much as possible.
- Close your eyes and concentrate on your body.
- Try to feel the tension flow out of you.
- Concentrate on parts of your body one at a time. It may be best to start with the legs and work up to your neck (often the site of most unrecognised muscle tension).
- First tighten up the muscles in each area and then relax them as much as you can.
- Concentrate on letting them go as floppy as possible. Feel the difference between your loose, relaxed muscles, and the tension required to tighten or move them.
- Imagine a probe going all round your body to seek out the tension and knots in the muscles and then relaxing them.
- Take deep slow breaths. Let your whole body and mind sink into a deep state of total relaxation.

Relaxation gets easier with practice, and there are lots of tapes, booklets and advisers willing and able to help you.

1. Keep you heels together and stretch your legs and toes. Then relax them completely.

2. Stretch out your arms and fingers. Hold them taut for only a moment before easing the strain completely.

3. Press your shoulders down on the floor. Then relax them.

4. Screw up your face muscles, and then let them relax.

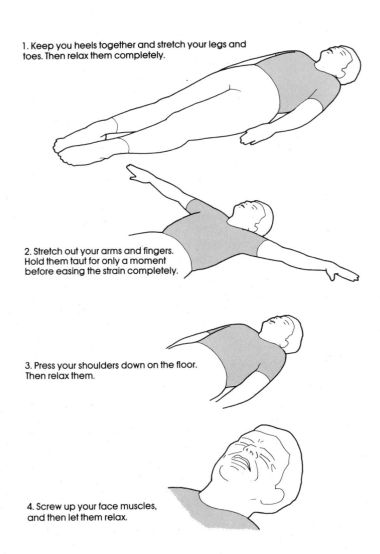

**Relaxation may be the most important skill you could possibly acquire.**

## Joint protection

Inflamed or damaged joints need respect and protection and the special advice or help of the occupational therapist. The objects of 'joint protection' are to reduce pain, conserve energy, reduce the risk of flare-ups of inflammation and help prevent deformity and damage occurring in your joints. It is common sense to look after your joints if you have arthritis, so the second rule of self-help is *respect and protect your joints*.

### Principles

The principles are fairly simple and obvious:
- Reducing mechanical stress on joints by spreading the load and doing things efficiently;
- Avoiding things that mean repeated stress on a joint or use of awkward positions;
- Interrupting periods of activity with rest;
- Generally looking after yourself.

### Some examples

- To protect hands – it is best to use two hands instead of one when lifting, to avoid too much heavy lifting or having to grip things tightly, and to use the palm and forearm to protect the fingers and wrists from too much stress.
- To look after shoulders and elbows – use lightweight bags or handbags, make sure your clothing is simple and easy to get in and out of, use long, sweeping movements of your arms instead of short sharp ones.
- Hips and knees – adjust the height of your bed, chairs and so on, so that they are easy to get in and out of, avoid standing for long periods, don't rush up and down the stairs unnecessarily.
- Feet – use lightweight shoes that support your feet but don't squash them. Avoid footwear that hurts, and try to avoid too much rushing around on uneven surfaces, as that puts a lot of stress on your feet and ankles.

## Rest and exercise

In general, exercise is much more important than rest but inflamed joints need rest, and during flare-ups of arthritis the whole body (and mind) may need a period of proper bed rest. It is vitally important, however, not to let joints get stuck or muscles waste – always do daily exercises so that you stay as supple and strong as possible. It is better to do a little too much than a lot too little! So the third rule of self-help is do *regular exercises for muscle strength and joint movement.*

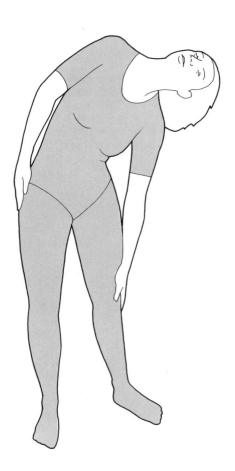

**Objectives**

The objectives of your regular exercises are:
- To maintain the full range of joint movement;
- To prevent deformities, and joints becoming stuck;
- To reduce pain and stiffness;
- To keep muscles strong (which also protects the joints).

A set of limbering-up exercises are useful for everyone and other specific exercises may be important, depending on the condition and which joints are affected.

**Limbering-up exercises**

These are best done first thing in the morning, either shortly before getting out of bed or before you get dressed. Work from your feet up:
- Work your ankles up and down and around in a circle as fully as possible;
- Bend your knees fully, and straighten them right out;
- Do the same for your fingers, wrists and elbows. Stretch your arms right up above your head;
- Roll your head gently from side to side.

Repeat each of these movements some 10 times, without rushing, so that you are fully loosened up before the day begins. If you have a lot of stiffness in the morning a warm shower or bath or exercising hands in a basin of warm water may help.

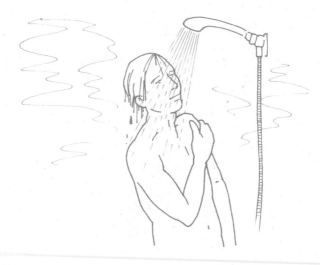

**Specific exercises**

It is particularly easy to let your fingers, shoulders or knees get stuck and weak. Here are some examples of exercises that can help prevent this:

- Knees – it is particularly important to keep the thigh muscles strong and to avoid them getting bent up. Sit yourself up in bed or in a good chair, straighten the knee fully and try to push it backwards (you will feel the thigh muscles tighten), hold it for a count of five and then relax. Repeat this 10 or 20 times for each knee.
- Hands – try placing them flat on a table, palms down, and 'walking' the fingers across to the thumb, as well as squashing the fingers and wrist flat. Bend your fingers right up into a tight ball, and stretch them fully.

Exercises are the speciality of the physiotherapists. You may need their professional help.

## Your home, garden, work and sport

Arthritis may mean that you can't do as much as you would like, that you can't do things quickly, and that you have to do some things in a different way. This doesn't have to mean that you stop doing things, however. The trick is to find ways round the problems, to limit the amount you do, and to intersperse periods of activity with rest breaks. You may need to plan your days and weeks carefully, setting aside rest periods, exercise and relaxation times in your routine.

### The home

You may need to think about the layout of your kitchen, bedroom and bathroom. You may need to use aids to help lift a heavy kettle, or open a jar or can, for example. The occupational therapist can help enormously in this area.

### Garden

You may need to make some adjustments in the garden too. For example, a light trug and a long-handled hoe can ease the weeding;

### Work

Positioning your desk and chair at work may make quite a difference to the amount of physical stress and abnormal postures you have to put up with each day.

### Sport

This needn't be a closed book to an arthritis sufferer either. Swimming, for example, can be an excellent, soothing exercise, and there are many clubs and organisations concerned with sports for disabled people.

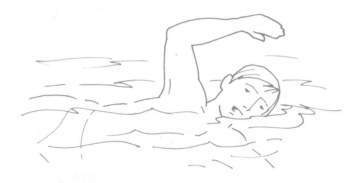

## Common questions and problems

Discussions about arthritis often bring up the same sort of questions. There is no good answer to some of them, but it may help to hear about the sort of things that often concern other people.

### Diet

There is no magic diet for arthritis. Diet doesn't make much difference to most people with arthritis. A few find that some foods, dairy products or red meats, for example, seem to make it worse, but there is no clear pattern to apparent food sensitivities. Fish oils and sunflower oil are being investigated for their ability to reduce inflammation, and dietary treatments are being researched. The most important thing for most people, however, is to keep on a balanced, normal healthy diet.

## The weather

Many people find that changeable weather makes their arthritis worse. Falls in barometric pressure seem to increase joint pain, and the pressure often drops just before rain. Weather has no long-term effects and you won't cure your arthritis by moving to somewhere with a different climate.

## Attitudes

It is often very difficult for relatives and for relationships to adjust to one person having arthritis. A spouse may be frightened, or try to deny the problem; others become overprotective. Sexual problems are not uncommon. Family relationships and patterns of behaviour are often strained.

Try to talk frankly and openly about all of these problems. If need be, consider asking for professional help, from a social worker or counsellor. There is nothing wrong with asking for help and talking things through often makes the answers obvious.

People with arthritis often feel that they are not understood. You may look fit and well, and others may not understand your feeling tired and not being able to do everything normally. Having arthritis has none of the glamour of some disorders, and it's often difficult for those around you to appreciate what's going on.

## Coping with tiredness

This is one of the most difficult battles for many people. Regular rest periods help, an hour on the bed in the middle of the day for example, but the continuous feeling of exhaustion is a real problem.

## Keep fighting

Many people get anxious about giving in to the disease and 'letting go'. It is often important to go on fighting, and it is crucial that you keep up your standards and appearance. That can be difficult. You need to learn new skills and find ways round the everyday problems. Again, being able to talk about it helps. Some people need to swallow some pride in order to be able to share their problems and get the help they need.

## Nobody understands

This is another common problem voiced by people with arthritis. In many ways it must be true; no-one who hasn't got arthritis can really understand. But many people, including doctors, are anxious and able to help. If you have a positive, outgoing attitude and if you can talk about it, you will find more understanding and help at hand. The problem for many doctors and their patients is to get over the feeling that they are supposed to be finding a 'cure'. Coping with arthritis is about caring, not curing.

## Coping with disability

Different people find different ways of coping. There are as many strategies as individuals. But some of the principles are the same, and most of the answers obvious, if difficult.

Accept all the help you can get: financial, medical and social. Look for ways round (not through) problems. Use your ingenuity. Adjust your goals and expectations to the possible. Keep as cheerful and active as you can, and don't withdraw from life. No-one is interested in the 'moaning minnie' who can't or won't help themselves, but there is endless help and sympathy for those who struggle with adversity.

Talking to and sharing the problems of people with severe, chronic arthritis has been a privilege and an education for me. I am constantly amazed, humbled and surprised by the cheerful way in which many people handle enormous problems. Sharing with others who have arthritis can be one of the best ways of learning how to cope.

# Useful addresses

**The Arthritis and Rheumatism Council for Research** 41 Eagle Street, London, WC1R 4AR (01–405 8572). The ARC finances an extensive programme of research and education and produces a series of helpful booklets on individual diseases which are available from the Council, your family doctor or rheumatologist. Other handbooks such as *Your Home and Your Rheumatism* can be purchased from the Council. It publishes a magainze, *ARC*, three times a year for the general public.

**Arthritis Care** 6 Grosvenor Crescent, London SW1X 7ER (01–235 0902/5). This is a welfare organisation that provides information, advice and practical aid to rheumatic sufferers. It has branches throughout the country and publishes a regular paper *Arthritis News* for its members.

**National Ankylosing Spondylitis Society** 6 Grosvenor Crescent, London, SW1X 7ER (01–235 0902/5). This is a society for sufferers from ankylosing spondylitis, their families and friends, and doctors and research societies working in the field. It aims to provide a forum for sufferers and to educate patients, the professions and the public in the problems of the disease. It produces a useful guidebook for patients and a 20-minute cassette tape of physiotherapy exercises.

**Back Pain Association** Grundy House, 31–33 Park Road, Teddington, Middlesex TW11 0AB (01–977 5474). The Association raises funds to support research into the causes and treatment of back pain and to help to alleviate and prevent back pain by teaching people to use their bodies sensibly. The Association also forms and supports local branches throughout the country to disseminate information and provide neighbourly help to sufferers.

**The Disabled Living Foundation** 380–384, Harrow Road, London, W9 2HU (01–289 6111). This was the first of the Disabled Living Centres. It is a national information resource service on any aspect of living with a disability. These centres concentrate mainly on aids and equipment for home use and give advice directly by phone and letter.

An aids and equipment centre is on site and can be visited by appointment. The Information Service is open 9.30 am–5 pm Monday to Friday (stamped addressed envelope appreciated).

There is an information sheet on osteoarthritis and rheumatoid arthritis *Ideas to Assist Those with Arthritis*, and a reading list is produced by their librarian.

**The British SLE Aid Group** 25 Linden Crescent, Woodford Green, Essex. Their role is in raising money for research. They distribute free booklets, pamphlets and information on lupus erythematosis both here and abroad to doctors and patients.

# Index

acceptance of arthritis, 28, 112-13
  *see also* attitude, positive
active arthritis, 26, 28, 44, 47-8
acupuncture, 108
ageing, 8, 16, 17, 23, 32, 84-5
aids and appliances, 37, 50, 89,
  99, 119-20
allergy treatments, 110-11
alternative complementary
  medicine, 89-90, 107-11
ankylosing spondylitis, 13, 17, 21,
  22, 53-8, 59, 68, 88
  and surgery, 102
  *see also* back
anti-inflammatory drugs, 38, 50,
  58, 59, 66, 67, 93-4
arthrodesis, 103, 105
articular disorders, 12-13
aspiration, 36, 59, 66, 67, 98
aspirin, 38, 66, 93, 94
attitude, positive, 26, 29-30, 50, 89,
  113, 121, 122
autoimmunity, 23, 24, 41, 69

back, 34, 44, 54-8, 105
  pain, 12, 16, 55-6, 79-82
  *see also* ankylosing spondylitis
blood pressure, high, 35, 63, 65,
  66
blood tests, 46, 47, 57, 66, 81
bone, 7, 9, 11, 42
  damage, 73
bursae, 10-11, 42, 64, 76-7

capsule, 10, 33
carpal tunnel syndrome, 79
cartilage, 9, 11, 13, 32-3, 64
causes
  of ankylosing spondylitis, 54
  of arthritis, 19-24, 73
  of back pain, 80
  of gout, 63
  of osteoarthritis, 32
  of periarticular disorders, 76
  of rheumatoid arthritis, 40-1
children and arthritis, 16, 83-4

chiropodists, 99
chiropractors, 89
codeine, 93
colitis and arthritis, 60
collagen diseases, 73
connective tissue diseases, 69-71,
  95
  mixed, 71
copper bangles, 111
cortisone, 94
counselling, 99, 121
crepitus, 35
crystals
  calcium, 35-6, 67-8
  as trigger, 13
  uric acid, 63, 64, 65, 66
cysts, 45, 104

defence mechanism, 23
  changes in, 16
deformity, 15, 44, 57, 84, 103
depression, 28
dermatomyositis, 71
dextropropoxyphene, 93
diet, 12, 22, 50, 87, 110
disability, 13, 15, 16, 25, 27, 29-30
  coping with, 122
disease-modifying agents, 95-6
d-penicillamine, 50, 96
drug treatment, 61, 66-7, 89, 91-8
  for osteoarthritis, 38
  for rheumatoid arthritis, 50
  side effects of, 46, 50, 60, 91,
    92-3, 93-4, 95, 96

effects of arthritis, 15-16, 24, 25-30
elbow, 44, 105, 116
  tennis, 12, 14, 79, 97
elderly, arthritis in, 84-5
environment as cause, 41, 54
exercise, 37, 48, 56, 57, 58, 78, 89,
  117-19, 120
eye inflammation, 56

feet, 33, 44, 105, 116
fibrositis, 12, 79, 84

fingers, 34, 35, 60
flare-ups, 44, 95, 98
fluid, 10, 11, 45, 47
  withdrawal of, 36, 59, 66, 67
frustration, 25, 28

genes as cause, 21-2, 32, 40-1, 54,
  58
gold, 50, 96
gout, 13, 16, 17, 21, 62-7, 95, 96
  prevention of, 66-7
  treatment of, 86
growing pains, 83
growth, 24, 84

hands, 33, 44, 71, 105, 116, 119
herbal remedies, 50, 110
hip, 33, 44, 85, 116
  replacement of, 39, 58, 103, 104
holistic approach to treatment,
  87, 91, 107
homoeopathy, 50, 109
hydrotherapy, 87, 108
hydroxychloroquine, 50, 70, 96

immobilisation, temporary, 81
infections, 13, 22, 72
inflammation, 24, 33, 35, 42-3, 45,
  54, 67, 69, 76
  of bursae, 11, 12
  of synovial membrane, 10, 13
injection into joints, 39, 50, 78, 95,
  97-8
injury as cause, 9, 12, 16, 22, 31,
  34, 64, 67, 76

joint
  effect of disease on, 33, 42,
    54-5, 64
  fibrous, 11
  infection in, 72
  locked, 28
  loss of function in, 27, 28
  number affected, 26
  and pain in children, 83
  and pain in elderly, 84-5
  protection of, 116
  replacement of, 39, 58, 103, 104
  scan, 36
  structure and function of, 9-11
  synovial, 9
  tumours in, 72

juvenile chronic arthritis, 17, 83-4

knee, 33, 44, 116, 119
  housemaid's, 12, 79
  replacement of, 39, 103, 104

ligaments, 10, 12

manipulation, 81, 89, 107
membranes, 10, 33
metatarsalgia, 79
movement
  importance of, 48-50, 117-19
  loss of, 28, 44, 54, 56
muscles, 7, 10-11
  spasm, 81
  strengthening, 37, 48, 117
musculoskeletal system, 7-11

neck, 16, 44
nodules, 42, 45

obesity, 22, 31, 35, 37, 63, 65, 66
occupational therapists, 39, 89,
  99-101, 116
orthotists, 99
osteoarthritis, 13, 16, 17, 21, 22,
  31-9, 103, 104
  and crystals, 67-8
  and effect on joints, 33
  nodal, 35
  people at risk of, 31, 35
  and surgery, 102
osteopaths, 89, 109
osteophytes, 33
osteoporosis, 80
osteotomy, 39, 103, 104
overuse, 12, 76

pain, 11, 12, 13, 14, 15-16, 24, 25,
  27, 28, 34, 43, 79, 83, 85
  back, 12, 16, 55-6, 79-82
  killers, 92-3
  relief, 38
paracetamol, 38, 93
Parkinson's disease, 84
periarticular disorders, 12, 14,
  75-9
  injections for, 97
physiotherapists, 37, 57, 78, 81, 89,
  90-101, 119
polyarteritis nodosa, 71

polymyalgia rheumatica, 17, 85, 95
polymyositis, 71
pseudogout, 17, 67
psoriatic arthritis, 59-61, 102
psychological damage, 46, 85
   in children, 84

Raynaud's phenomenon, 70, 71
reactive arthritis, 58-9
reflexology, 111
Reiter's syndrome, 58-9
relaxation, 114-15
remission, natural, 86, 108
rest, 48, 70, 77, 78, 81, 89, 117-19, 121
rheumatism, 11, 14
rheumatoid arthritis, 13, 21, 22, 23, 40-52
   people at risk of, 17, 40
   and surgery, 102
rigidity of spine, 54
risk of arthritis, people at, 14-18, 31, 35, 40, 54, 58, 63, 69, 76, 80, 83, 84

scleroderma, 70
self-help, 112-22
sex, effect of, 16-17
shoulder, 14, 44, 85, 105, 116
   frozen, 79
sicca syndrome, 71
side effects of drugs, 46, 50, 60, 92-3, 93-4, 95, 96
Sjorgren's syndrome, 71
slipped disc, 80, 81, 105
spine *see* back
steroids, 70, 85, 94-5, 97
stiffness, 27-8, 34, 43, 54, 55, 79, 85
sulphasalazine, 50, 96
surgery, 39, 89, 102-6
   types of, 102-3
swelling, 35, 42, 43, 45, 83
symptoms
   of ankylosing spondylites, 55-6
   of arthritis, 27-8
   of back pain, 81
   of gout, 64
   of osteoarthritis, 34-5
   of periartiular disorders, 76-7
   of reactive arthritis, 59
   of rheumatoid arthritis, 43-4
   *see also* pain; stiffness; swelling
synovectomy, 103
synovium, 10, 13, 33, 44, 64, 103
systematic lupus erythematosis, 69-70, 95

tendons, 10-11, 12, 42
tension, dangers of, 114
tests
   for ankylosing spondylitis, 57
   for back pain, 81
   for gout, 66
   for osteoarthritis, 36
   for periarticular disorders, 77
   for rheumatoid arthritis, 46-7
therapists, 48, 50
   *see also* occupational therapists; physiotherapists
thumb, 34
tiredness, feelings of, 28, 121
toe, 34, 60, 63, 64
treatment
   of ankylosing spondylitis, 57
   of arthritis, 86-90
   assessment of, 48
   of back pain, 81
   drug, 91-8
   of gout, 65, 66
   holistic approach to, 87, 91
   of osteoarthritis, 37-9
   of periarticular disorders, 78
   of psoriatic arthritis, 60
   of reactive arthritis, 59
   of rheumatoid arthritis, 48-51
   surgical, 38, 89, 102-6
   types of, 88-90
tuberculosis, bone and joint, 72
tumours in joints, 72
types of arthritis, 11-12

ulceration, 45
urine tests, 47, 66

warmth, use of, 87, 88, 99, 108
weather as cause, 22, 120
wrists, 44

x-rays, 36, 46, 47, 57, 58, 66, 81